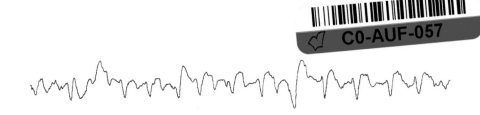

# SAVING JESSE

## A Diary
## of
## Rasmussen's Syndrome

*by* Nicky Armstrong
*with* Jeanne Heal

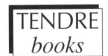

TENDRE
*books*

Design and layout by Donald Ward
WARD FITZGERALD EDITORIAL DESIGN
314 – 1121 College Dr
Saskatoon SK  S7N 0W3


Printed and bound in Canada


**Canadian Cataloguing in Publication Data**

Armstrong, Nicky, 1957 –

Saving Jesse, a diary of Rasmussen's Syndrome

ISBN 0-9681373-0-X

1. Armstrong, Jesse – health.   2. Chronic encephalitis – Patients – Saskatchewan – Biography.
I. Heal, Jeanne, 1947 –     II. Title.

RC390.A74 1996    362.1´96832´0092    C96–920148–6




Tendre Books
2416-2nd Ave. N.
Vanscoy SK  S0L 3J0

# Contents

# Foreword

Rasmussen's Syndrome is a rare brain disease that was described for the first time in 1958. Dr. Theodore Rasmussen and his colleagues described three patients who underwent operations for uncontrolled epilepsy. The surgery was performed in the Montreal Neurological Institute. Pathological examination of the epileptic brain tissue showed findings of inflammation. This suggested that the cause of the disease was an unusual viral infection. Recent experimental evidence suggests it may be due to an autoimmune process, an inflammatory disease in which the body treats its own tissues as foreign.

The disease affects primarily children and leads to progressive loss of brain tissue in one cerebral hemisphere. The clinical result is intractable epilepsy and a progressive weakness of one side of the body.

This book describes a boy who went through all the stages of Rasmussen's Syndrome. He was the first patient—in fact the only patient in my practice—with this rare disease. With Jesse and his family, my knowledge of the disease has evolved and grown; physicians have much to learn from their patients. The author, Jesse's mother, describes clearly her fears and her anxieties. She writes of her efforts to seek the best possible treatment for her child and of her trips across Canada and the United States to famous medical institutions, always looking for answers and possible treatments.

Eventually Jesse and his family were faced with the major decision of undergoing a destructive operation where the diseased cerebral hemisphere is removed. The book discusses the effect of such a prospect on the family and friends of Jesse and describes how the community became involved and supported the family through their difficulties.

This book demonstrates an understanding of the medical, social, and personal aspects of a very serious brain disease. It will be of wide interest to people involved in the health care of children, as it displays how the life of a normal six-year-old can be altered totally by disease, how the family react, and how doctors, nurses and others struggle with difficult issues, sometimes with knowledge but often in ignorance. It shows how these parents were faced with a very difficult decision for their child's ultimate welfare and how in this case their decision was ultimately correct.

Noel Lowry, MD, FRCP (C)
Pædiatric Neurologist
Royal University Hospital
Saskatoon

# A Personal Word

During my son Jesse's five-year illness I kept a daily diary. At first my purpose was to keep track of the seizures—their nature and frequency—to help the doctors reach a diagnosis. As the disease progressed and Rasmussen's Encephalitis (or Rasmussen's Syndrome, as it is now more commonly known) was diagnosed, I continued the diary in the hope that some of this information would aid in finding a cure. Later I kept the diary in order to some day tell our story. This diary is the basis of *Saving Jesse*.

Although there is still no cure for this debilitating condition, there is a treatment. Hemispherectomy, although a radical procedure, is in our experience the only effective means of putting a final stop to the deterioration of our children.

I urge those families with children who suffer from idiopathic seizures to continue their search for a cause. Don't stop until you're satisfied that you've investigated all avenues and exhausted all options. Medicine is always advancing; knowledge is always expanding; new treatments are continually possible. Never give up hope.

To those families with children who are now diagnosed with Rasmussen's Syndrome, I urge you to keep up with advances in its treatment and thoroughly research your options. The more you learn, the less fearful you will be—I know this from personal experience. Always be hopeful. There is life after Rasmussen's Encephalitis. Jesse is proof. I wish you strength and compassion in your quest.

Nicky Armstrong
Vanscoy, Saskatchewan
November 1996

# Acknowledgements

I wish to thank the following people and organizations who have been instrumental in bringing *Saving Jesse* to publication:

Hoechst Marion Roussel Canada Inc., Laval, Quebec, for their generous financial assistance.

My sister, Jeanne Heal, for her encouragement and her writing skills which enabled her to condense and clarify my rough draft into a clear and concise story, bringing it to life.

Donald Ward, for his excellent editorial skills and his instant faith in this story. Thanks for making a good story better.

On a more personal note, I am indebted to:

Chris, my husband, for listening to me, understanding me, and loving me.

Tara, my daughter, to whom this book is dedicated. I am proud of the young woman you have become.

Dr. Noel Lowry, Pædiatric Neurologist, for his continued guidance and support.

Doris Newmeyer, Nurse Co-ordinator, for your encouragement and optimism.

Dr. Robert Griebel, Neurosurgeon, for your compassion and expertise.

Dr. John Freeman, Professor of Neurology and Pædiatrics, for sharing your knowledge and maintaining your priorities, putting the interests of the children first.

Diana Pillas, Co-ordinator-Counsellor, for your support, and for your determination to gain the best quality of life for "your kids."

My mom and dad, my sisters and brother and their families. I am grateful to all of you, for your understanding, your support, and your love.

The Armstrong family. The miles between us are many, but we always felt your presence, especially in the dark times.

All my friends, especially Bev Turgeon, Faye Sanders, Shelly Bolianatz, and Barb McLachlan. Thank you for your endless support. I could always count on you.

Cindi and Steven Binder in Colorado and Brian and Kathy Usher in Connecticut, parents like us, for your understanding and your message of hope.

There are many others I wish to thank: Henriette Morelli, Melissa Morelli, and Myrtle Ebert for reading the manuscript and offering suggestions and encouragement; the Kinsmen Foundation; The Children's Wish Foundation; the Royal University Hospital E.E.G. staff; everyone who took part in the Jam for Jesse, the Vanscoy Hockey Tournament Fundraiser, and the Vanscoy Elementary School Pancake Breakfast; the Delisle Community Chapel; the Delisle Elks Club; Agrium Inc. (Potash Operations); Ed, Ivy, and Danielle in Montreal; and others too numerous to mention who uplifted and supported us with a kind word or deed. You have all touched our lives.

And of course Jesse, for your love of life, your agreeable nature, and your positive attitude.

Guess what?

I love you.

With love to my daughter, Tara,
for her courage and compassion.

# 1 / A Symptom, Not a Cause

Seven AM, November 7th, 1986. My eyes flew open at the sound of a child crying. I threw off the blankets and ran toward the sound. I found my five-year-old son, Jesse, standing unsteadily in the bathroom. He was clutching his abdomen.

"What's wrong, Jesse?" I asked, kneeling beside him. "What's the matter?"

He didn't look at me. "It hurts," he moaned. His words were slurred and distant, as if he were speaking through a cloud of pain. He seemed almost unaware of my presence.

"It hurts," he moaned again, still clutching his abdomen.

I took his face in my hands and looked into his eyes. They weren't Jesse's eyes. They were far away and glassy. He continued to moan and whimper with the pain. I didn't know what was happening to him. I only knew Jesse wasn't seeing me at all, and I was afraid. I called my husband, Chris. Together, we tried to talk to Jesse and comfort him, but he didn't respond to our voices, couldn't tell us what was wrong. We tried to sit him on the toilet. Maybe it was just a touch of the flu, I thought, or gas pains. There was nothing we could do but stay with him until it was over.

The incident, the attack—whatever it was—eventually passed. It seemed an eternity, but the pain subsided, and Jesse returned to normal. I could see it in his eyes: wherever he had gone, he was back now. Chris and I tucked him into bed. When the family got up for breakfast, Jesse was fine. That was obvious from looking at him. He didn't remember getting up in the night, and he didn't remember the pain.

All that day I tried not to think about it, but I couldn't shake a feeling of uneasiness. I mentioned the incident while I was visiting my parents later that afternoon. They had raised six children, and there wasn't much that could surprise them.

"It was probably nothing," Dad reassured me in his comforting Quebecois accent. "You know kids. They walk in their sleep. You used to walk in your sleep—and talk, too."

I wanted to believe him. But the feeling of uneasiness stayed with me.

A week later, *it* came back. It was early morning again, only this time I was awakened by our four-year-old daughter, Tara, calling Jesse's name. I found Jesse on his bedroom floor, crying and holding his stomach.

"Jesse, what's wrong?"

He mumbled something I couldn't understand.

I spoke louder: "Jesse, look at Mommy! What's wrong?"

He could only murmur and moan. I looked into his eyes. They were glassy and unfocused. He wasn't there.

Close to panic, I scooped him up and ran to our bedroom. His body was limp one moment, rigid the next. I put him on the bed, where Chris and I talked to him as we had before, trying to comfort him, or just to reach him. There was no response. But gradually, as before, he stopped whimpering. The stiffness left his body, and he fell asleep. I watched him, holding my breath, waiting for something else to happen. His body twitched occasionally. Other than that, there was no hint that anything might be wrong. He woke up an hour later as if he had spent the night in peaceful sleep.

"Jesse, do you remember being sick last night?" I asked, trying to sound nonchalant.

"No," he said, puzzled by the question.

"You had a stomach-ache in the night. I think I'll keep you home from kindergarten today, just to make sure it doesn't come back."

But Jesse loved school, and he wasn't feeling the least bit sick. "Please, Mom," he pleaded. "I really want to go to school. I'm okay. Honest."

I watched him as he got dressed, ate his breakfast, brushed his teeth. At the first sign of something—anything—amiss I would take him to the doctor. But there was nothing. He was my Jesse again. So I gave in and let him go to school.

It was my bowling day. I dressed Tara for the cold November weather and we drove to Saskatoon with Sandy, a neighbour and friend. All through the game, I worried about Jesse. I wanted to phone the school, but I kept telling myself I was paranoid. Jesse was fine. And I'd be home in less than an hour.

As soon as we finished bowling, I called my doctor's office and spoke to the nurse about Jesse's episode. I wanted her to say, "I'm sure it was nothing, if he's all right now." Instead, she said, "You should bring him in to be checked, just to be certain."

We live in Vanscoy, a small town ten minutes west of Saskatoon. The drive back that day seemed to take hours. I asked Sandy to drive me to the school so I could check on Jesse. The principal, Barry Grosse, met me as I walked in the door. He said, "Mrs. Armstrong, Jesse had a seizure."

My heart went cold. "A what?"

"Jesse had a seizure in the gym at about eleven o'clock."

How could he tell me that and look so calm?

"What are you talking about?" I asked sharply. "How is he? I want to see him."

"He's fine. We called Mrs. Turgeon"—Bev Turgeon was a close friend and neighbour—"and she said she'd take him to the minor emergency clinic. He's with her now."

My mind was whirling. I'd never seen a seizure. I hardly knew what they were. But I had to get to Jesse. I had to look into his eyes.

Jesse's teacher was waiting for me in the kindergarten room. We sat at a child-sized table on child-sized chairs. The alphabet danced across the wall in bold colours while I had a surrealistic conversation about my son.

"We were in the gym," Mrs. Johnstone told me, "in a circle, holding hands and singing, when Jesse let go of the children's hands. He began to weave. At first I thought he was fooling around. I pulled him toward me, but he was unsteady, and fell down." She paused. "Then he began to convulse. His eyes rolled back, and his arms and legs bent. It lasted about a minute. Afterwards he was sleepy and disoriented. We called Mrs. Turgeon and she came to pick him up."

I heard the words, but they barely registered. Suddenly I didn't like her. I didn't like the school. I didn't like these people who could tell me so casually that my Jesse had had a seizure.

"I've got to go to him," I said, and the little chair I'd been sitting on toppled over as I stood up. I rushed out to the car. "Jesse's sick," I told Sandy. "He's at Bev's." In a whisper, I added, "They said he had a seizure."

Sandy drove directly to Bev Turgeon's. On the way there I had time to be thankful that Jesse was with her. If there was anyone I could count on, it was Bev. I first met Bev about a week after we had moved into the trailer court, in June 1986. She walked over one day in the rain, looking like a mother goose with three wet ducklings. She said she had been lonely when she first moved into the trailer court, with her husband Lyle working at the mine nearby. She didn't want a new neighbour to feel the same way. From that moment, she was like a safety net below a tightrope. She was always there for me.

As the car pulled up, I jumped out and ran into the house without ringing the bell. "Where's Jesse?" I demanded. "Is he okay?"

Bev put a hand on my arm. "Don't worry, he's fine. They checked him out at the minor emergency clinic, and told me to take him home." She pointed to where Jesse was lying on the couch, watching cartoons. "See for yourself."

I ran to him. "Jesse?"

He turned to me, love and recognition in his large brown eyes. "Hi, Mom."

Bev was right, he looked fine. I hugged him tightly. He didn't say anything, but I could tell he was puzzled by this burst of smother-love. I looked again for some evidence of what had happened. It had left not a mark on him. Yet I knew, now, that it would come again. I didn't know when, or why. I didn't even know what it was. Ignorance breeds fear, and I was scared as hell.

The minute we got home I was on the phone to the doctor's office.

"Bring him in to emergency at St. Paul's Hospital," I was told.

I called Chris at work. He came straight home and we took Jesse to the hospital. Tara stayed behind with Bev.

Jesse didn't know what the fuss was about. We told him he had been sick at school and we had to take him to the hospital. He didn't remember being sick at school, but he went along with it, easygoing and cheerful, as always.

We drove to the hospital in silence. I was afraid to ask Chris what he was feeling. If he wasn't as frightened as I was, then maybe I was wrong about the severity of Jesse's condition. But if he was terrified, too, then I didn't want to hear about it.

We arrived at the hospital around 3:00 PM. I began to fill out the forms, the first of many times I would perform this task. Date of birth, place of birth, length of labour....

Jesse was born in Calgary on January 24th, 1981. It was a long and difficult labour. After thirty hours, he was finally delivered by Caesarean section: a healthy nine-and-a-half-pound baby boy.

Shortly after Jesse was born, the economy took a down-turn in Calgary. Chris had to go to Edmonton to find work, coming home on week-ends. We had purchased our first house only a few months before. We put it on the market, but with interest rates hovering around 21% there weren't many buyers. In September, the house still unsold, Jesse and I moved to Edmonton so we could be together again as a family.

Jesse was a bright and beautiful little boy. He walked at nine months, and he spoke early, too. He was toilet trained at twenty months—just in time for the arrival of our daughter, Tara, who was delivered by Cesarean section on October 8th, 1982.

The week before, the house in Calgary finally off our hands, we had moved into a new home in Bon Accord, a community a few miles north of Edmonton. The economy was still in a slump, though, and work in the construction industry once again was slow. After a year, we found ourselves unable to meet our mortgage payments. Instead of waiting for a repossession notice, we simply gave the house back to the bank, along with the equity we had built up over the years. We weren't alone. Four other families in the neighbourhood—some of them middle-aged couples who had been there for years—had to give up their homes and start over.

It was a hard decision, but it seemed the only sensible choice. Chris and I packed up our family and moved to a mobile home in Vanscoy, ten minutes outside Saskatoon. For me, it was like coming home. I was born and raised in Saskatchewan, and my parents, four sisters, and my brother all lived in the province. It was different for Chris. He was from Richmond Hill, now a suburb of Toronto. He'd been on his own since he was sixteen. His main concern was to find work and support his family.

I continued filling out the medical form:

> Has the patient ever been hospitalized? *Tonsillectomy when he was two and a half.*
> Has the patient or an immediate relative ever had heart problems? *No.*
> Polio? *No.*
> Dizziness? *No.*
> Chest pain? *No.*
> Epilepsy? *No.*

In the examining room, the resident went over the questions with me, then admitted Jesse for further testing to determine what had caused the seizure. Once Jesse was settled, he was eager to find the play room. He didn't seem to mind that he had to stay in the hospital, or that he had to have a needle. All he wanted was to find the play room.

His attitude was a blessing; I was worried enough for both of us. While he was in the playroom, I went to find a phone. I dreaded having to talk to my parents and the rest of the family. I had been comforting myself with denial, but now I would have to admit, out loud, that Jesse had had a *seizure*. How I hated that word. In the end I called my mother and asked her to let the rest of the family know. Then I called Bev Turgeon. I managed to maintain my composure until I hung up. Then I sat in the phone cubicle and cried.

While Jesse was in the hospital he had a CT scan and several blood tests. After four days, Chris and I met with the neurologist, Dr. Siemens. The results were in, he told us. Everything was normal. He handed me a prescription: "This is for Phenobarb, an anticonvulsant. It's only a precaution," he added, seeing my hesitation. "It will calm the brain in case there's a tendency to seizure. We recommend it whenever anyone has seizures and we can't determine the cause."

Chris asked, "You mean, Jesse's going to have more of these . . . seizures?"

The doctor shrugged. "He may, or he may never have another. Some people don't have any more after the initial one."

Summoning all my courage, I asked the unthinkable: "Could . . . could Jesse die?"

"Death from seizure is so rare as to be negligible," he replied.

Slowly, I took the prescription from him. "What do I do if he does have another one?"

"Time it. If it continues past three minutes, bring him to the hospital."

On the way home I made the first of many desperate pacts with God: "Please let my Jesse-boy be okay. Don't let him have another seizure. I'll do anything you ask, if only you make it go away."

Over the next week we monitored Jesse's every move. We were always on edge. Chris's thirty-first birthday came and went on November 20th, but it was completely uneventful. Jesse was all we could think about. On the 25th he had his first electro-encephalogram at University Hospital.

The EEG records electrical impulses in the brain. Twenty-two coloured wires were attached with paste and gauze to designated spots on Jesse's scalp. At the end of each wire was a metal electrode which fed information back to the machine. The process was not painful, but Jesse hated it. He couldn't stand the stench of the ammonia they used to dissolve the glue that kept the electrodes in place on the scalp. He never complained about the hundreds of injections he received over the years, or any of the other painful procedures he had to endure. But he dreaded the EEG.

On November 27th, Chris was out of town on business when Jesse had another seizure. For the first time, I saw it for myself. I was wakened at 6:30 AM by a noise in the bathroom. I didn't even think. I ran. Then I saw him. My Jesse, my baby, down on the bathroom floor, his legs twisted, his face contorted, his whole body jerking with each spasm.

*My God!* I thought in horror. *What am I going to do?*

I caught a movement in the corner of my eye, and turned toward it. Tara was standing in the doorway, her eyes wide as she stared at her convulsing brother. I shut the door and yelled at her to go away. Her brother was going to die, and I couldn't let her see it. *Protect him, protect her,* I thought.

*Don't let her see. She's only four years old. It will terrify her for the rest of her life.*

I spoke nonsense to Jesse, my voice shaking, reassuring him, asking him if he could hear me, telling him it would be all right. I kept babbling as I looked at my watch. *I have to time this. If it lasts more than three minutes. . . .*

It lasted, in fact, about a minute. It felt like an eternity.

I scooped him up. My hands were trembling and my legs felt like rubber. I laid him on my bed. I asked him if he was okay, and I kept asking until I got an answer. I had to know he was still there, that Jesse was still alive in this limp, dragged out, little boy's body with the saliva dribbling from his lips.

Finally, he whispered, "Yeah."

I got his coat on over his pyjamas, then I dressed Tara. I took her to Sandy's, then drove to St. Paul's Hospital with Jesse. On the way, I kept talking to Jesse. He was desperately tired, but I couldn't let him sleep. *If he's talking,* I reasoned, *he can't die.*

When we arrived on the ward, a resident came to ask all the same questions I had answered the last time.

"Has he been exposed to chicken pox?" he asked, finally.

"Yes," I said. "His sister came down with chicken pox a week or two ago."

*Is that what caused this? Chicken pox?*

"I'm sorry," the resident said. "I can't admit him."

I was taken aback. "You have to. He's sick. You have to find out what's wrong with him."

"I'm sorry," he said again, shaking his head. "I don't have the authority."

"Then, please, get someone who does."

The head of pediatrics was a thin, tactless, middle-aged man. "I cannot admit your son," he told me, "because he has been exposed to chicken pox. I will not risk an epidemic on the ward."

"But he had another seizure," I pleaded with him. "I saw it myself."

He was unimpressed, but I wouldn't give up.

"You have to find out why he's having these seizures," I insisted. "You can put him in a private room if you don't want to expose the other children, but I'm not taking him home."

The doctor was adamant. This was his ward, his responsibility, his empire. I was told to leave. With no choices left, I stormed out of the room and took my son with me.

As before, he seemed to recover fully, with no ill effects. But a week later, he called me from his bedroom: "Mom, I can't move my head off the pillow."

"What do you mean?"

There was no other way to put it; he could not move his head off the pillow. I made him try again, but his head and shoulders seemed to be pinned to the bed. It lasted only a few minutes, but he was left with a headache.

I worried again—still—more. But this time I got angry. *What the hell's going on here?* I demanded. *What will happen next? Somebody had better make it stop!*

I called my doctor. He told me to take Jesse to St. Paul's Hospital. They were going to do another CT scan to compare to the last, but this time they would inject a dye into his body which would darken the densest areas of his brain so that any abnormalities would be more prominently displayed. It was called a "contrast." The technician assured me it wouldn't be painful. "The worst anyone feels is a warm sensation as the dye is injected," he said.

I watched. Jesse lay on a sliding table top designed to move millimetre by millimetre through a plastic, doughnut shaped apparatus. With each millimetre the table advances, the scanner films a slice of the patient's brain until an image of the entire organ was formed.

His head rested in a U-shaped holder, with sponges by his ears and straps on his forehead to keep him immobile. His body was also strapped in. It was imperative that his head not move while the pictures were taken. When he was secured to their satisfaction, they found a vein in his arm and injected the dye.

Jesse immediately began to heave and thrash about. His face went pale. Everyone watched in silence. Then someone pulled the straps off Jesse's head. Someone else brought a basin, so he could vomit.

"What's wrong?" I demanded, trying to suppress the panic in my voice. "What's going on?"

"Some people are allergic to the dye," the technician explained. "It's very rare. Your son is displaying a mild reaction."

*Mild?* I wanted to scream at him. *This isn't just "some people!" This is my Jesse! He's only five years old!*

Jesse was calmer than I was. He didn't get upset, he didn't cry. He just accepted it as something he had to do. The technicians proceeded with the scan and we were sent back up to the ward.

I discovered later that there is a non-allergenic dye, but the hospital didn't like to use it because it was much more expensive. From then on I insisted that Jesse get the non-allergenic dye. Sometimes I met with resistance, but by then I had learned how things were done. I made it clear that either he got the dye that didn't make him sick, or the procedure would not go ahead.

Jesse stayed in the hospital three days this time, and he was given his first lumbar puncture, or spinal tap. I knew nothing about the procedure except that it was extremely painful. The patient assumes a fetal position, arching his back to stretch the discs of the spinal cord, and then a needle is inserted between the discs to withdraw some of the cerebrospinal fluid. This is the same fluid that surrounds the brain inside the skull.

Again, I was assured that Jesse would be fine, but after the experience with the dye, I wasn't so sure. I wanted to be with him while the procedure was being done. I was told that was not possible. It wasn't allowed: "But don't worry. There will be other people in there to help him along."

*If it's not allowed, it's not allowed,* I reasoned, and let it go. After they had taken Jesse out to the examining room, I decided to go down to the cafeteria. When he returned he would have to lie flat for several hours, so this would be my last chance for a coffee for a while.

As I walked to the elevators, I heard Jesse's voice, shrill and frightened, coming from down the hall. *"No, no!"* he was screaming.

I couldn't go to him. They had told me I couldn't be with him. It was not allowed. But how could I stand there, helplessly listening to him scream?

I punched the button for the elevator. It didn't come and it didn't come, and still I could hear Jesse's fear and pain.

The elevator still didn't come. Finally, I couldn't stand it any more. *God, help him!* I pleaded, and ran for the stairs. I ran all the way down, and when I reached the bottom, tears were streaming down my face. I vowed I would never again allow this or any other procedure to be carried out unless it was in my presence.

When the results were in—the CT Scan, the spinal tap, all the blood work—I was told that everything appeared normal. Something terrible was happening to my child, and no one could find out what it was.

A month after Jesse's first seizure we began to notice a change in his personality. I thought it was the medication. He was becoming hyperactive on the Phenobarb, so the neurologist suggested he change to Depakene. Finding the correct dosage took weeks, and countless blood tests. Then one night I was sitting on the edge of his bed, ready to say goodnight. He began to recite his prayers—"Now I lay me down to sleep"—but he had forgotten the words.

"Jesse, don't be ridiculous," I scolded. "You've been saying this prayer since you were two years old."

But he wasn't joking. He couldn't remember.

On December 28th, Jesse had another seizure. We rushed him to the hospital. Again he was examined and released.

We met with the neurologist, Dr. Siemens, on January 8. Jesse's first CT scan, he told us, had revealed a possible hypodensity in the right frontal lobe of Jesse's brain. In the second test, the brain appeared normal. Because the two results were contradictory, he had ordered another scan for next week. In the meantime, we were no further ahead—although Doctor Siemens did tell us that he had only limited experience with children. The only pædiatric neurologist in Saskatchewan was Dr. Noel Lowry. Fortunately, he practised in Saskatoon. An appointment was arranged. In the meantime, Jesse had another CT scan. The results were normal.

That same day, my father was admitted to the hospital with a blood clot in his leg. He had a history of poor circulation, and was often in pain. I visited him in the emergency ward for a while, then took Jesse down the hall for his scan, then returned to emergency. Dad never complained, but I could tell by looking at him that he was suffering. Mom didn't leave his side. He was scheduled for bypass surgery on January 20th. On that day, the family was informed that the surgery had been a success. Dad was in intensive care, but he seemed to be recovering well.

The next day, we were told that he was slipping in and out of a coma, and he had developed another blood clot. The following day he was worse. His legs were blue and cold from lack of circulation. He was developing pneumonia.

Five of his six children were at the hospital with Mom, who left only when she needed to sleep. The surgeon spoke to all of us. He said the only possible way to give Dad more time would be to amputate. It was a terrible decision. We asked the surgeon what he would do if it was his father. He said, frankly, that he wouldn't amputate. With pneumonia setting in, there was little chance Dad would survive the surgery; if he did, there would be terrible pain. He was seventy-six years old. He had always said he would rather die than lose one of his limbs. Our decision was unanimous.

We took turns at his bedside in the Intensive Care Unit. When it was my turn, my sisters warned me that he didn't look like himself. I walked cautiously to the side of the bed, and gave Mom a hug through her tears.

Dad's face was grey and swollen. He looked older than I had ever seen him. But it was still him, and he was still my father. I took his hand, and Mom said, "Nicky's here." Eyes closed, he gave my hand a little squeeze. He knew. My main concern was that he wasn't in pain. Throughout our lives he had made each of us believe, somehow, that we were his favourite. I thought he was the last person in the world who deserved to suffer. I asked Mom, and she spoke into his ear: "Dad, are you in any pain?" With his eyes still closed, he mouthed the word, "No."

We were at the hospital on and off the next day. That night I woke up in a cold sweat. Moments later, Jesse woke up and vomited. The phone rang. Dad was slipping away. I should come to the hospital. I called my brother, Ernie, who lived a few miles away, and told him I would pick him up. As I was getting dressed, the phone rang again.

"Nicky, Dad just died."

Ernie and I drove to the hospital, where we went in to say our final good-byes. He was disconnected from the machinery and looked very peaceful.

It was January 24th, 1987, Jesse's sixth birthday.

A few days later we were visiting Sandy and her husband, Konrad. It was late afternoon and our children were playing happily in one of the bedrooms. Then Tara came into the kitchen and said, "Mom, Jesse won't talk."

Chris and I both ran. Jesse was sitting on the bed, staring, jerking a bit. I called his name, but there was no response. I picked him up and held him on my knee. He wasn't convulsing, but he wasn't with us, either.

*What is happening to him now?*

I called again: "Jesse, look at me!"

Still no response.

"Jesse, look at Mommy. Can you see Mommy?"

At one point he drawled, "Yes," but he wasn't looking at me. His body was stiff, but his head was limp and his eyes were glazed. We put on his coat and took him home, where Chris laid him on his side on the bed. He was spitting up, mostly saliva. He hardly moved. He looked wrung out. I called the neurologist, then we rushed Jesse into Saskatoon. In the car Jesse told me he had a headache. Then he fell asleep.

At the hospital, the doctor determined that Jesse had an ear infection. We were sent home with a prescription for antibiotics.

Throughout February of that year, Jesse had different types of seizures. He would stare, unresponsive, for thirty to sixty seconds. Sometimes he would drool, and sometimes he would pick at his clothing; sometimes he did both. He was exhausted afterward, and would usually fall asleep. One day he came into my room and said his left arm felt funny and was hard to move. At this point, nothing seemed strange. I had been keeping a record of each seizure—date, time, and duration—to see if there was a pattern. So far, I had learned only that anything could happen at any time.

On February 25th, we drove into the city for our appointment with Dr. Lowry. We were understandably anxious, but our expectations were high. We thought we would finally be getting some answers. We arrived at Royal University Hospital, and with desperate confidence made the trek from the parking lot, up the elevator, and through the long overhead walkway.

In the waiting room we kept a close eye on Jesse, as we had been doing for the past few months. Doris, Dr. Lowry's nurse, took us into the examining room. She was lively and personable, and her air of confident optimism helped allay our fears. She introduced us to Dr. Lowry.

We would come to know Dr. Lowry as a kind, gentle, good-humoured man whose eyes sparkled with lively interest whenever the conversation turned to new methods of treatment or neurological procedures. But when we first met him, our minds and hearts were full of Jesse. All we saw was a tall, thin man with long, artistic fingers. He spoke with a slight Irish inflection.

He examined Jesse thoroughly. He performed the neurological tests with which we would soon become familiar:

"Walk in a straight line, heel to toe. . . . Jump on your left foot. . . . Good. Jump on your right foot. . . . Good. Now close your eyes, put your arms out, and touch the tip of your nose with your pointer finger. . . . Now touch my finger, then your nose. Again. . . . And again. . . . Good."

To Jesse it was all a game to please the doctor. When Doris took him to the playroom and returned alone, I began to worry. Jesse was never left alone any more. What if he were to have a seizure?

Dr. Lowry told us that the results of his neurological examination were normal. Then he told us that Jesse had epilepsy. I reached for Chris's hand. This was bad. I wasn't sure what the word meant, but this was very bad. I began to cry. How could he so matter-of-factly tell us that our child had epilepsy? It suggested a permanent condition. Before this word was uttered, Jesse had only suffered a few seizures—which would go away, surely.

I didn't know at the time that "epilepsy" is just another word for "having seizures." I didn't know it was a symptom, not a cause. Chris and I were dejected as we walked out of Dr. Lowry's office with a copy of *Does Your Child Have Epilepsy?* I made sure no one could see the cover of the book as we picked Jesse up in the playroom.

I expected him to look different, now that he had epilepsy. He didn't. He looked the same as always.

# 2 / Status Epilepticus

It was only after I arrived home and began reading *Does Your Child Have Epilepsy?* that I rebelled against the diagnosis. I read the section on "What is *not* epilepsy?" with hope, trying to fit Jesse's spells into one of the categories. To no avail. The book also spoke of the many possible causes of epilepsy, but none of them seemed to apply to Jesse. I had been hoping to find some answers. I found plenty of them, but not the one I was looking for: how to make the seizures go away.

"Low potassium can cause a seizure," I read. Maybe that was it. Over the next few weeks, I fed Jesse bananas until he couldn't bear the sight of them. Then I thought maybe he wasn't getting enough sleep, so I made sure he slept more than any normal six year old.

He had had a concussion when he was two years old. Maybe that was it. The doctor at the time had said it was a slight concussion. He'd be fine; just watch him for the night. But maybe he hadn't been fine.

Maybe it was a food allergy. I took him to an allergist. He was allergic to dust and cats, neither of which would indicate seizures.

When he had his first seizure, I remembered, his sister and many other neighbourhood children had had chicken pox. Jesse didn't get them. Did something go wrong there? We didn't know. Neither did the doctors.

In the meantime, Jesse's personality continued to change. The open-hearted and joyous child I'd spent so much time with when Chris was working in Edmonton was becoming impulsive and demanding, and his memory was deteriorating. In the book it said that, except for the seizures, there is no difference between people with or without epilepsy. Seizures alone do not cause brain damage. Yet I knew something inside my son was changing.

In April, I registered Jesse for his first year in T-ball. He loved playing ball, and I turned up dutifully to watch him. I never volunteered to keep score; Jesse might have a seizure and I would have to go to him. Sometimes I was asked, and I didn't like to refuse. But I always managed to keep my eyes on Jesse.

He didn't have any seizures while playing ball that first season. But they didn't go away. He had one in April, one in May, and another in June. We were always on edge, waiting for the next one, dreading its arrival, and praying to God that it wouldn't come—or that it would be the last. We always held to that hope. When a few weeks went by without a seizure, our hopes would soar. But they were always knocked down with a thud. Then we'd pick them up and start over again.

I found comfort in the Bible, and I began to retreat to my bedroom in the evening to read it. A passage from Luke, particularly, I read over and over:

> On the next day, when they had come down from the mountain, a great crowd met him. And behold, a man from the crowd cried, "Teacher, I beg you to look upon my son, for he is my only child; and behold, a spirit seizes him and he suddenly cries out; it convulses him till he foams, and shatters him, and will hardly leave him. And I begged your disciples to cast it out, but they could not." Jesus answered, "O faithless and perverse generation, how long am I to be with you and bear with you? Bring your son here." While he was coming, the demon tore him and convulsed him. But Jesus rebuked the unclean spirit, and healed the boy, and gave him back to his father. And all were astonished at the majesty of God (9.37–43).

I read everything I could find on epilepsy. I spoke to anyone who knew someone who had epilepsy. And I prayed for faith and healing.

From the time medication was first prescribed, I hated the whole idea of it. Jesse was only a child; a little boy shouldn't have to be taking drugs. Nevertheless, by May I was giving him Depakene three times day—at 8:00 AM, 4:00 PM, and 8:00 PM—as the doctor had ordered. But most of his seizures occurred in the morning. If the doses were equalized over a twenty-four-hour period, I reasoned, Jesse would have enough Depakene in his system to prevent those morning seizures. I called Dr. Lowry's office. Doris listened patiently. It was not necessary to administer anticonvulsants that way, she said, but it couldn't hurt. I set to work at once, giving Jesse his medicine at precise, eight-hour intervals, even if it meant waking him up at midnight. It wasn't many weeks before I realized what Doris had known all along: this wasn't the answer, after all.

$B$y summer, Jesse spoke of having "bad thoughts." He couldn't explain them, but he had also been experiencing muscle twitches more or less constantly. I knew that these and the "bad thoughts" were connected to the seizures.

Lately, Jesse was becoming nauseous after his seizures. He sometimes vomited, and often had a severe headache that would last from two to four hours. The pain was so bad he could only moan; it hurt too much to cry.

Chris and I shared our own pain in silence. Like my father, Chris was never one to talk about his feelings. He was dealing with himself. I was trying to deal with myself. Poor Tara was lost somewhere in the middle. I kept thinking, *When Jesse gets better, I'll devote more time to Tara. When Jesse gets better, I'll lose some weight. When Jesse gets better, I'll stop smoking. When Jesse gets better. . . I'll live again.*

Not surprisingly, I was having nightmares. I woke up one night in a cold sweat, crying so hard that Chris woke up, too. I couldn't stop. But I couldn't share the grisly details of the dream with him, either. I just kept crying. He gave me a hug, and I was eventually able to calm down enough that he could get back to sleep. But every time I shut my eyes, the nightmare returned. It consolidated all my fears.

I had an enormous fear of losing Jesse, physically: he'd be having a seizure and I couldn't find him. I was also afraid that, when he was alone, convulsing on the ground, a dog would attack him and I wouldn't be there to protect him. I was even more afraid of losing the inner Jesse, his beautiful soul. And I was afraid of losing Chris somehow; I was afraid that if something happened to Jesse, Chris wouldn't be able to carry on. He wouldn't be there for us.

The dream brought all these fears together: Jesse was outside playing, but when I called him, he didn't answer. I searched for him frantically. It was growing dark, and I was still looking. I sensed that he was close, possibly having a seizure. I saw a hole in the ground. Every instinct told me not to look, but I knew I had to. I bent down slowly and peered in. There were gophers the size of rabbits, gnawing on something with their buck teeth. Bones. I knew in an instant that they were eating my baby. I screamed, then I ran. I couldn't get home fast enough. I opened the door and bolted through the porch, calling Chris's name. My sister Henriette stopped me at the kitchen door. She grabbed me and held me back. I kept calling for Chris, but he didn't come. Henriette didn't say anything, but her eyes told me that they already knew about Jesse. Chris was lost to himself in a dark room. He had gone out of his mind when he found out. In that instant I knew I'd lost them both. I let out a bone-chilling scream. That was what awakened me.

Later, I resented Chris for not being supportive enough to me during those hard times, resented him for not opening up to me. I wanted him to be a pillar of strength. I wanted him to be my confidante. Yet, at the same time, I didn't want to hear about his fears. I wanted him to tell me that everything was going to be all right. Perhaps his silences were his way of coping, but he may also have been trying to protect me. He knew that the words, "Tell me how you feel," really meant, "Tell me how you feel, as long as it's positive." Because of his inability to express his feelings, I felt he was not supporting me. Paradoxically, it was because of this same inability that I considered him my pillar. It was a struggle working it out alone, for both of us.

We could not have managed without the support of family and friends. A couple of times a year, one or another of my sisters would offer to look after the kids for a few days so Chris and I could get some time alone to catch our breath and mend our courage. As for friends, there was Bev Turgeon.

Bev was of average height, but slim, with shoulder-length hair that made her look taller. She had three boys and is only a year younger than I, but many people mistake her for a teenager. Often salespeople who came to the door would ask to speak to her mother. She and Lyle had married young, and were happy in their marriage.

Also that summer I met Faye, who was enthusiastic and full of energy, with a cheery personality. She worked during the day, so I saw less of her than I did of Bev. Her two children were involved in numerous activities, so Faye seemed to be forever on the go. Still, I always knew she was only a phone call away.

On July 2nd, Chris and I drove Jesse to Prud'homme to stay with my sister Yvonne, her husband David, and their three girls while Tara visited Henriette and her husband, Eddie, for a few days. I gave Yvonne instructions about Jesse's medication, and what to do if he had a seizure.

"The likelihood of anyone going into a seizure and not coming out of it is extremely small," I told her, "although people have been known to suffer brain damage, or even death, if they're left too long. If he goes into a *grande mal* seizure for longer than three minutes, take him to the hospital." I told her again that the chance of this happening was almost nonexistent, but I wanted to make sure she knew what to do in any eventuality. I could tell she was uneasy, but she assured me everything would be fine.

About fifteen minutes later, on the highway to Saskatoon, I started to panic. I had never believed in premonitions, but at that moment I knew something was happening.

"Something's wrong," I said. "We can't leave Jesse."

Chris thought it was just the normal anxiety of letting him out of my sight. There was that, it's true, but this feeling of dread sent a chill through me.

I knew that my sisters were capable, responsible people. They had only our interests at heart when they insisted that they take the kids for a few days to give Chris and me a chance to be alone. They knew what a strain Jesse's illness had put on us, and thought it would be good to give the whole family a breather.

We drove on.

I called Yvonne that night. She said everything was fine. I called again the following day, and again everything was fine. "No sign of a seizure," she said. I breathed a sigh of relief. It was then I decided to relax and make the most of the time I had away from the kids. I made plans to go shopping with a friend the next day. I was up early and getting ready when the phone rang. Yvonne's voice was close to panic.

"Jesse's in a seizure!" she said. "I don't know what to do."

I spoke slowly, my voice reassuring. "Is he in convulsions?"

"Yes," she said, "I woke up at 8:00 to give him his pills and he was on the floor. The bed was wet and—Oh Nicky!—he's still in the seizure!"

Only a minute or two had gone by since she had found him. I was frightened, but I spoke calmly: "Turn him on his side so he doesn't choke. He should come out of it shortly. Call me back as soon as he's done. He'll be okay."

I hung up and waited for what seemed an eternity, but in fact it was about three minutes. Then I called back.

"Nicky, he's not coming out of it!"

She was supposed to say, "He's fine now, but it scared me." After all, the chances were so slim. At least, that's what they had told us. People rarely go into *status epilepticus*.

"Take him to St. Paul's Hospital," I told her. "We'll meet you in emergency." My voice was urgent, but I tried to hide my fear. "I'll let them know you're on your way." Again I reassured her: "He's going to be okay."

I was sure he wasn't going to be okay, but it was the only thing to say. I dialled the hospital emergency ward. A doctor there told me I should tell them to go to University Hospital, which was closer, but when I called back, they had already left. While Yvonne and David rushed Jesse to the hospital, their three girls were on their knees with a neighbour, praying that Jesse wouldn't die.

Chris and I jumped in the car and headed for the city, a fifteen-minute drive. We made it in no time. It took an eternity. I spoke to myself all the way. Jesse would be out of the seizure by the time they got to the hospital. After all, it was a twenty-five minute drive from Prud'homme, then another twenty minutes to St. Paul's. When the panic welled up, I started the process again: Jesse would be out of the seizure by the time they got to the hospital. . . .

Chris was silent.

We parked the car and ran into the hospital. Jesse wasn't there yet, but they were prepared for his arrival. The minutes ticked by. We paced. We waited. We scanned the streets for Yvonne and David's car. Finally they arrived. Chris and I ran out and opened the car door. Yvonne had wrapped Jesse in a blanket, with his head to the side and facing down so that his airway was clear and the saliva could run freely from his mouth. He was still convulsing softly. He was pale. His eyes were blank. He looked lifeless.

Chris scooped him up and ran back through the hospital doors. A nurse took him, and they immediately started an intravenous of Valium and Dilantin to stop the seizure. We waited anxiously. Soon he began to respond. It was only then that I really saw Yvonne. Her face was strained and pale, her eyes wide. She was terrified. "I'm sorry," I kept saying, "I'm so sorry," as if it were my fault. But if this had to happen, I wished it had happened at home. It was my cross to bear, not hers.

The four of us huddled together and waited. It wasn't long before we were ushered into a separate room. The doctor spoke calmly, but chose her words carefully. Jesse was out of danger, she said, but we couldn't be sure if he had suffered brain damage until he was awake and responsive.

I stood at Jesse's side with Chris. Our small son was in a deep sleep. His colour looked good. I held his hand and spoke to him gently. I wanted him to wake up and speak to us, but I was afraid, too. Had the thief left without a trace, or had he scarred this innocent life forever?

The doctors kept him under observation for a while. Chris and I observed him somewhat more intently. How could a body endure such violence and remain unaffected? It seemed unthinkable, yet as Jesse slowly responded to my questions, I knew he would be all right. Even so, when the doctors decided he was stable and could be discharged, I insisted that they admit him and observe him overnight. They did as I asked. There were nocomplications and no further episodes.

On August 19th we had another appointment with Dr. Lowry. The CT scan from the previous week showed no change from those of last November and December. The doctor now concluded that all the CT scans showed a small, hypodense area in the right frontal lobe. Although Dr. Lowry could not be 100% sure, he thought it likely that the area in question represented old scarring from a previous injury.

If that was scar tissue, I thought, then Jesse would have to live with seizures and medication for the rest of his life. Would his personality continue to change? If so, then the old Jesse was gone. In either case, his life would never be normal.

"Could it be a tumour?" I asked, almost hopefully. *They can remove tumours*, I reasoned, *and then he would be okay.*

"Believe me, Mrs. Armstrong, you don't want it to be a tumour."

Guilt and resentment flooded over me, in equal measure. Of course I didn't *want* it to be a tumour. I didn't *want* any of this! I had simply thought that a tumour might be the lesser of two evils.

Doctor Lowry continued: "We'll repeat the scan in another six months with a contrast. I'll review him again in early September."

He spoke so casually that I couldn't help thinking that he considered Jesse's case rather commonplace. If that were so, why couldn't he fix it?

Two days later, Jesse was running a fever. I took him to our family doctor to make sure he didn't have an infection. He didn't. But later that evening he went into convulsions. I called for Chris, praying that this seizure wouldn't be like the last one. *Please let it end*, I prayed, as we timed it for two tense minutes. Time seems to stand still when you have to watch your child convulsing. A two-minute seizure seems to stretch to ten, even twenty, so actually timing it helps you keep a sense of proportion.

When it was over, I gave him an aspirin and let him rest. I checked on him every fifteen minutes for the rest of the evening. By 11:00 PM his temperature still hadn't come down. We got him dressed and took him to the hospital. An emergency room doctor diagnosed a throat infection and wrote out a prescription for antibiotics. As we waited, Jesse slowly turned his head and began to stare, his face twitching slightly. I recognized it immediately as a seizure. The doctor said he couldn't be sure. I was sure. I asked that Jesse be admitted for observation in case he had more seizures, for a high fever might increase the chances of his going into status again.

"All right," the doctor said. "I'll admit him as soon as I have a minute."

The doctor didn't have a minute. As far as I could tell, he was the only doctor on the ward. We waited and waited. Jesse was still awake. There were no more signs of seizures. By 3:30 AM, exhaustion overcame fear. We took Jesse home.

I knew all about fevers. When Jesse had gone through a bad year with recurrent bouts of tonsillitis, I had slept with him, checking his fever every hour. I gave him Tylenol. When the Tylenol didn't bring his temperature down, I gave him cool baths. I set up a makeshift air conditioner—a bucket of ice on a chair with a fan blowing across it—to keep the air cool. Knowledge, patience, persistence, and love—they always beat a fever.

Seizures were another matter. They snuck up on you. They struck without warning. The parent who must watch and wait helplessly has no more control than the child who must endure it. With Jesse's seizures out of control, my life felt out of control.

# 3 / Setting New Limits

In September 1987 Jesse began grade one and Tara was enrolled in Kindergarten. I made arrangements for the school to call Bev Turgeon if something happened and I should be unavailable. If I was away from home for any length of time, I called Bev periodically to see if the school had phoned. She made it clear it was no inconvenience, but I know there were times she cancelled her own plans just so she would be there. I tried not to take advantage of her generosity.

Jesse had learned to ride a bicycle the previous summer, and had ridden it to and from kindergarten before his seizures began. Now he was six years old and in grade one, but there were new limits to set.

"Can I ride it after school, just around the trailer?" he pleaded.

We finally agreed that he could ride it around our mobile home if I was outside watching him. This didn't last long. There were no accidents, but I decided it was just over the edge of the "too dangerous" category.

Jesse had a few more episodes of what he called "bad thoughts." Increasingly, he also had that other type of seizure—I called them "absence seizures"—where he would turn his head and stare vacantly, his body twitching. After we added Tegretol to his medication, the bad thoughts diminished. But the absence seizures began to increase. Whereas previously he had been having one or two a month, in September he had twenty-five or thirty. They lasted anywhere from fifteen seconds to two minutes, and when they were over he would often fall asleep.

The myoclonus, or muscle jerks, were evident day and night. Often I would sit at his bedside with my hand on him. Every few seconds his arm, leg, head, hand, or foot would twitch. It looked as if these were tiny seizures trapped inside, trying to get out. I thought he must be uncomfortable with all this inner activity, yet he seemed able to sleep. He also moaned in his sleep, which he had not done before the seizures started.

In September Dr. Lowry did a blood level test and checked Jesse neurologically. I asked him if patients on anticonvulsants routinely had as many seizures as Jesse.

"Yes," he said, "there are some patients with idiopathic seizures—seizures we don't know the cause of—and the medicine doesn't control them. But," he quickly added, "they would have many more attacks without the medication. Sometimes we have to experiment with different medications, or different combinations of medications, to find the right one for each individual."

I was slightly less afraid of Jesse's seizures than I had been a year ago, but they still frightened me. If Jesse was silent for more than five minutes, one of us would casually check on him, or we'd call his name. If he answered, we would say, "Nothing." If he didn't answer, we'd call again as we ran to him. Even Tara started doing it. If we heard a bang or an unusual noise, we would run toward the noise. The tension was almost unbearable, even for Jesse. One day, exasperated, he asked, "Why does everybody call me, and then when I say 'What?' you say 'Nothing'." We learned to back off—not relax, but back off.

One evening, just after we had put him to bed, he came down the hall, screaming. Chris and I both bolted up at the same time. Jesse came into the living room, yelling, "My tooth! My tooth fell out!" We laughed with him as our heartbeats slowly returned to normal.

On September 21st I spent the morning with my brother, Ernie. Jesse was in school and Tara was at kindergarten. At noon we stopped in at my sister Jeanne's house, where I was going to call Bev to see if the school had phoned. Jeanne met me at the door.

"Bev called," she said. "Jesse's had an accident. He's at St. Paul's Hospital."

My heart jumped. "Is he okay? What happened? Did he have a seizure?" But Jeanne didn't have any details. *He must have had a seizure,* I thought. *But if he's in the hospital he must be in status. No, not that again!*

My anxiety was all-consuming. My mind flooded with scenes of the last time he'd gone into status: doctors hovering around the gurney, prodding, poking, trying to stop the convulsions that wracked his body. *You had no right to go away today,* I scolded myself. *You have a sick child. You should have been at home.*

Ernie was a step behind me as I rushed through the hospital doors. We met Bev and Lyle coming out. They had called Chris, who was already waiting inside.

"Is he okay?" I gasped. "What happened?"

"He'll be fine," Bev reassured me. "He fell off the monkey bars. They think he must have had a seizure. His face is swollen, but they took an X-ray and it was okay. He's inside with Chris."

"Thank you," I said, and hugged her. "I'm sorry. . . ."

She waved me off with a smile. "Forget it."

I was completely unprepared for what I saw when Jesse turned to me. His big hazel eyes seemed tiny in his swollen face. It was hard to tell where his cheeks ended and his nose began. His upper lip was cut, and three times its normal size.

"Hi, Mom," he said. "I had an accident."

"You sure did. Are you okay?"

He swung his left arm and said, "Yeah, but my arm hurts a bit."

If Jesse said he was fine, you couldn't be sure. But if he said something hurt, it definitely did. I asked for an X-ray. Sure enough, there was a hairline fracture in his wrist. We waited as they made a cast over his hand and up to his elbow.

The next morning he got up early to watch cartoons, as he usually did. About half an hour later, Tara came into our room and said that Jesse wasn't talking to her. "He was shaking when I got up and he wouldn't answer me," she said. I bolted out of bed and ran to the living room. He was still in a seizure, his eyes staring. I put him on the couch and asked him questions. For fifteen minutes there was no change. He was able to understand and answer, but his responses were slow, almost mechanical. Finally, the vacant look left his eyes, and he fell asleep.

Later that day, he was standing at the kitchen table reading to me when suddenly he stopped. I called his name. There was no response. He began to turn his head to the left. Slowly, his body followed, but his feet stayed firmly planted. When he could turn no more, he moved his feet, then continued turning to the left. I spoke to him, but he didn't respond. He made three partial revolutions this way—head, body, then feet—before I picked him up and sat him on my knee. He continued turning on my lap as I anxiously dialled Dr. Lowry's office.

"This is Mrs. Armstrong." My voice was high and urgent. "I need to speak to Doris Newmeyer. It's an emergency!"

In the short pause that followed, Jesse began to stiffen. The turning had stopped, but now he was starting to shake and jerk. He was going into convulsions. It felt as though I were holding someone else—some*thing* else, not a child, not even a person, certainly not my son. I put him down on the carpet, quickly, roughly, anxious to get this strange, unfamiliar child off my lap.

Dr. Lowry's nurse spoke calmly into the telephone: "Hello."

"Doris!" I screamed. "He's in convulsions!"

"How long has he been in the seizure?" she asked, articulating each word carefully.

"A couple of minutes." My voice was shaking. I kept my eyes on Jesse as I spoke. His body was jerking uncontrollably, the cast on his broken wrist thumping against the floor. "He started by turning to the left, like a robot. . . . Doris, it's not stopping!"

"Calm down, Mrs. Armstrong. He'll be fine."

She was right, of course. Within moments the convulsions began to diminish. Doris said to bring him in to the office. When we arrived, Jesse was extremely tired. Dr. Lowry examined him and said he would arrange for more blood tests and possibly increase the medication. When we got home, Jesse was so groggy that he fell in the hallway. I put him to bed and he slept for hours.

"Children with epilepsy are normal and should be treated normally."

So we had been told. But how could we treat Jesse like other children? How could we let him climb things, knowing any moment he could drop to the ground in a seizure? How could we let him ride a bicycle, knowing that he could fall off at any time, or steer into the path of an oncoming car? How could I leave him in the bathtub while I answered the phone? How could we let him use a knife, or hold a sharp object, when he might fall into a seizure and injure himself, even kill himself? How could we let him play outside after a rain? It takes only an inch of water in a puddle to drown a baby; Jesse in a seizure was more helpless than a baby.

I began to feel impatient toward my friends. Whenever they mentioned the problems they were having with their children, I thought how trivial they were. They complained about how their kids wouldn't phone to let them know where they were, or they wouldn't show up on time for supper. *If you only knew how lucky you are,* I thought, *not having to worry every minute they're gone, but only when they don't show up on time.* When they complained that their kids were hard on their bikes, I wished Jesse could just ride his. I was envious and angry that they didn't appreciate these things. They took their children's health for granted. I didn't have that luxury.

After Jesse fell off the monkey bars, the school recommended making them and the swings off limits to him. I was reluctant to agree to this, as I didn't want to make his world totally sterile and boring. I had asked him if he remembered the incident. He told me he had been hanging upside down, with his knees wrapped around one bar while he held on to a lower bar with his hands. Another child had pried his fingers off, and that's when he fell. I passed on this information to the school: Jesse hadn't fallen because of a seizure. If it had been a seizure, he wouldn't have remembered how it happened. Moreover, he hadn't gone into convulsions afterward, nor did he fall asleep, which always happened after a seizure.

I was met with scepticism. They couldn't be sure it *wasn't* a seizure, and there was always the possibility of a seizure at another time. I could understand their position, but I was afraid this was the thin edge of the wedge. Once a limitation was in place, they would have licence to institute others. Soon there would be limits on every situation, every action or activity in which Jesse wanted to take part. Had they suggested supplementary measures, such as increasing playground supervision, I would have been more receptive. But since Jesse didn't fit into their mould, they would whittle him down until he did. I wanted them to strike a balance, putting Jesse's best interests first.

One day soon afterward, I watched through the patio doors as Jesse stood on the deck waving goodbye to his father. He was walking toward the car, still waving. He kept walking and waving, and he was getting awfully close to the steps. Suddenly I realized he was in a seizure. He wasn't going to step down; he was going to keep on walking. He looked like a robot, walking and waving, even though the car was now gone. I ran out and grabbed him just as he was going to step into space. I led him into the house, talking to him all the while.

"Jesse, are you okay?"

"Now I know the reason," he said, slowly.

"What do you mean?" I asked, in some excitement. "The reason for what?"

I thought he had been given the answer, perhaps in some sort of spiritual experience. Maybe God was speaking to him, telling him why these things were happening to him. But he didn't respond. He was still in the seizure. When he came out of it he was groggy, as always, and fell asleep. When he woke up, I asked him again what he had meant, but he remembered nothing. After that, I reluctantly agreed to having his activities at school restricted.

Both Jesse and Tara were early risers. As early as 5:30 one or the other would call from their bedroom, "Mom, can I get up now?" I would turn over in bed and check the time. Anytime before 7:00 I considered still night time.

Jesse was the first caller at 6:30 one morning. "Mom, can I get up now?" "No," I called. "It's still night time. Go back to sleep."

When 7:00 rolled around, it was Tara's turn: "Mom, can I get up now?"

I was still tired, but 7:00 was morning. "Okay," I said, and I went to get her up.

When I went into Jesse's bedroom, he was still sleeping. This was unusual, especially as Tara and I had been calling back and forth. I let him sleep, but checked on him fifteen minutes later. He was in deep sleep; he was warm; he was alive. *Please God,* I pleaded, *don't let him be having seizures while he's sleeping.*

I went back to his room a few minutes later. He woke up, but he was groggy, and very like he always was after a seizure. I hoped I was wrong. I could be there for him during the day. The school could be there for him when he was at school. The baby monitor my sister Henriette and her husband Ed had given us could alert us to any cries in the night. But short of watching him all night, I couldn't be there for him if he was having seizures in his sleep. I tried to brush it off. I told myself he was probably just overtired. Some things I didn't have to face just yet.

A few nights later Tara called me in the night for a drink of water. After I got it for her, I went into Jesse's room. He was a light sleeper, and I knew he'd be awake and want a drink, too. Sure enough, his eyes were open. I asked him if he wanted a drink of water.

No response.

I asked him again. Still no response. He lay there staring, his eyes glassy, his left arm twitching. He was swallowing repeatedly. It lasted about three minutes, then he closed his eyes and he fell back asleep.

I would have to face it now: Jesse was having seizures in his sleep, and there was nothing I could do for him.

I hated it when the phone rang during the day. Each time I held my breath and hoped it wouldn't be the school. Each time they called, I'd say, "I'll be right there," then I would run. Sometimes they called while he was still in the seizure, and I'd pray on the run that he'd be out of it by the time I got there.

I had asked them to call me with each seizure, and I would come to school and pick him up. By the fall of 1987, however, the days Jesse had absence seizures began outnumbering the days he didn't. We had to change the arrangements. Now they called me only after a *grande mal.* The time and duration of each absence seizure was written down and sent home to me every day so I could keep track of them.

*Note sent from school, October 13th, 1987*

I was on supervision outside, at the far end of the playground when a student came running to tell me Jesse was "lying on the ground and can't hear anything." I ran to the far side of the school yard and Jesse was lying, partly on his side, on the grass by the school. His legs and arms were twitching and his breathing was in short, gasping breaths. His eyes were partly opened, but didn't appear to be focusing and his mouth was partly open.

I immediately sent a student in to tell Mr. Grosse to phone Mrs. Armstrong. The convulsions lasted 2–4 minutes while I was there. When they subsided, Jesse was very disoriented. I carried him inside and laid him down. His eyes were fluttering and rolled back. He was mumbling and had some saliva coming out of his mouth. (I noticed this when I picked him up outside.) He kept rubbing his forehead as if he had a headache. Mrs. Armstrong then came to get him.

On October 21st I took Jesse to the hospital to get his cast removed. They took another X-ray. His arm had healed perfectly. Two days later I took him in again, this time for a blood level test. His seizures were not getting any better. They were getting worse, even with the increased medication. I called Dr. Lowry. He said he would add another anticonvulsant, Rivitrol, to Jesse's medication.

I began this medicine on Monday night. By Tuesday morning, Jesse couldn't walk without bumping into walls and furniture, and his speech was slurred. It was as if he was drunk. He was extremely tired and slept for a few hours, not because of a seizure but because of the cure for the seizure. I phoned Dr. Lowry and told him what was happening. He said to reduce the dosage for a few days, then increase it slowly. This helped, but Jesse was still tired and slow. He looked drugged now instead of drunk. For the next ten days, he was seizure free—a walking zombie, but seizure free. Was this something to celebrate?

I spoke to Jesse's teacher. She said he was tired in school. It took a great deal of effort for him to answer questions, and she had to repeat instructions two or three times before he understood.

I reduced the dosage further, but it didn't help, and the seizures returned. Dr. Lowry suggested adding Dilantin, another anticonvulsant, to his medication. A few weeks later I spoke again to Jesse's teacher. She said he was changing rapidly. He had trouble remembering things, was disruptive in class, and pushed the other kids so he could be beside her at story time. And he continued to have seizures.

I saw the changes at home, too. He was increasingly forgetful, and he demanded constant attention. I was finding it difficult to like him. And that made me furious. I wanted my baby back. This child wasn't Jesse.

Notes from school were universally negative. I heard about the bad days or I heard nothing at all. It was time to try a new approach. The school and I agreed that, from now on, the teachers would send notes home only when Jesse had a good day. This way I, too, could reinforce the positive, and he was delighted when I praised him for having a good day. He always wanted to please. When he had a bad day now, he was crushed.

I asked Dr. Lowry about discontinuing the Rivitrol. Jesse's body did not seem to be getting accustomed to the drug. He was still dopey, distractible, and forgetful, and we weren't achieving much better seizure control. He agreed to increase the Dilantin and gradually reduce the Rivitrol until Jesse was off it completely.

*Diary entry, December 19, 1987*

Jesse had another seizure today at about 2:00. He was sitting on the chair and his head turned to the left. He said "what" when I called him, but couldn't answer any more. It lasted for about one minute.

I cut ¼ pill of his Rivitrol out this morning. Now he's just on ¼ in the evening. I increased his Dilantin this morning also. Now he's on 1½ morn, 1 at 4:00 and 1½ evening. He is also still on Tegretol, 3 morn, 3 afternoon, and 3 evening. I'm sick and tired of this crap. Nothing is going to work.

I felt Dr. Lowry was driving me around in circles, handing out increases and decreases and changes in medication to pacify me, all at Jesse's expense. We were living in hell and the Jesse we had known was dying before our very eyes.

On December 31st, Jesse was anxious to be up, as Yvonne and David and their three girls were visiting. They'd slept over, and were still scattered on the couch and floor in the living room in sleeping bags. I gave Jesse his morning medicine and went back to the bedroom to get dressed. All of a sudden I heard a huge bang. Instantly, Yvonne yelled, "Nicky!"

I ran to the living room. Jesse was in convulsions. Yvonne was holding him to keep him from falling. She said he'd been showing the girls something in a book when all of a sudden some invisible force seemed literally to throw him into the plexiglass stormwindow. He immediately went into convulsions. Yvonne was visibly shaken. The girls were upset also, remembering when Jesse had gone into status at their house.

I took Jesse and laid him down on the floor with his head to the side. I yelled, "Time!" for someone to time the seizure, and I kept repeating, "He's going to be okay." To Jesse, I said, "Honey, it's going to be okay. It's going to be over soon. You're going to be okay."

Within two minutes the convulsions had subsided. Jesse was tired, but this time he didn't sleep. Chris lay on our bed with him for about an hour. Jesse lay very still, but he stayed awake. When he got up he didn't have a headache and he didn't vomit. He was hungry and wanted breakfast. It was the first time he hadn't suffered any adverse effects from a *grande mal*.

# 4 / "They're Going to Fix my Brain"

We began 1988 with high hopes that Jesse would be healthy again. But on January 3rd he suffered another seizure, on January 4th another, and on January 6th yet another. He was off Rivitrol now, and his behaviour seemed to take a turn for the better, but he was still impulsive and he was still forgetting things.

Dr. Lowry had suggested that he ask Dr. Sundaram, who worked in adult neurology, to have a look at Jesse. He called on January 8th to tell me that his colleague had agreed to see Jesse. He also reported that Jesse's Tegretol level was still low, so we increased the dosage.

In the middle of January, I noticed Jesse watching TV with one eye shut and his head tilted to the side. "Everything looks double," he explained. "If I close one eye, it helps."

"How long has this been going on?"

"A few days." He didn't seem concerned.

That night Chris awoke with a start. Jesse was in the hall, swaying to the left and bumping into the wall. Chris helped him to the bathroom, then brought him to bed with us.

At the end of the month, Jesse's teacher reported that Jesse told her he was seeing double. He was starting to forget the letters of the alphabet, too.

Dr. Lowry put it down to the increase of Tegretol in his medication: "We'll cut it back and then increase it slowly and try to get it in the therapeutic range."

I argued that therapeutic ranges were only averages. Some people whose levels were testing at below the therapeutic range might actually be at the highest doses their bodies could handle. I suspected this was the case with Jesse.

Every phone call, every visit to Dr. Lowry was like a boxing match. I read everything I could get my hands on that might pertain to Jesse's ailment, then confronted the doctor with it. He invariably defended his actions, and we ended in a stalemate. I suspect he didn't likehearing from me. To be fair, I did call often. I had to. He was not only the most knowledgeable pediatric neurologist in Saskatchewan, he was the only one. I needed him.

*Diary entry, January 29, 1988*

Jesse had a seizure at 8:00 while he was eating breakfast. He just stared and moved his hands around for about a minute. He was tired afterward for a few minutes and his words were slurred, as usual.

The teacher phoned me at noon and said Jesse had another seizure in gym at about 11:50 that lasted for about two minutes. She said his eyes fluttered and went back a bit. He was tired afterwards and she put him to lay down, but he didn't want to stay. She said it was like yesterday's absence seizure, except his eyes didn't flutter as they did now.

Jesse's getting very forgetful and dozy again. It seems like he can't remember anything. His speech seems to be getting worse. He's not doing well in school. He can't remember any instructions. It seems life is just passing him by. He seems to be getting more and more immature. . . . I don't see much of a future for him right now.

A week later, Jesse's teacher called to tell me he couldn't keep up any more; she was sending him to the resource room for extra help.

When it was time for the next blood level check I didn't care about the results. I was determined not to increase any of the medications. Jesse was already a walking zombie. They would have to try another way.

One bright moment in that dismal month came on January 28th when Jesse was invited to a birthday party. It was the first party he had been invited to since kindergarten. When the seizures began, invitations stopped. He was anxious to go to this one.

I went to pick him up after school. While he was getting his things out of his locker, he went into an absence seizure. I bent down and held him on my knee. The after-school commotion was all around us: kids talking and laughing, getting ready to go home. No one noticed us. When the seizure passed, Jesse was tired, as usual, but he didn't want to go home and sleep. He told me in a drunken but determined voice that he was going to the party. I wondered then how many seizures the school had missed. They couldn't be with him every moment, of course, but it saddened me to think of the times he must have been alone.

On February 5th we brought Jesse to our appointment with Dr. Sundaram. He was dopey that day, as he had been for some time now. He didn't have the energy to jump about and be distracted. He just sat on my lap, his head on my shoulder.

Dr. Sundaram was soft-spoken and genuinely interested in helping. As we discussed Jesse's history, we agreed that his seizures had been at a minimum while he was on Depakene. He suggested re-starting the Depakene and tapering off the Dilantin. Then he said, "I recommend Jesse have an MRI scan to give us a clearer picture of the brain lesion. Unfortunately, we don't have an MRI in Saskatchewan, but Winnipeg, Vancouver, and Montreal each have one."

We were desperate for anything that might help. "Can you make the arrangements?" I asked.

"Certainly. There is something else you should keep in mind," he added. "Brain surgery is often performed on people whose seizures are caused by scars. Removal of the scars is often successful in arresting the seizures."

We were taken aback. As desperate as we were, brain surgery seemed too drastic. We had to take things a step at a time, and the first step was to determine the nature of the lesion.

By the middle of March Jesse was off Dilantin and taking Depakene and Tegretol instead. We continued to go for blood tests. His seizures did not diminish in number or intensity.

*Excerpt from Dr. Sundaram's report to Dr. Lowry, February 8th, 1988*
This patient's seizures might very well have right frontal origin. They are certainly proving intractable.

I feel an MRI scan is in order to assess the nature of the right frontal lesion. . . . Eventually we may have to consider further telemetry monitoring if the above medication changes do not work.

I felt vindicated, seeing it written down: the seizures *were* intractable.

At the end of February another type of seizure developed. We were playing cards, one of the things Jesse enjoyed that was not dangerous, when his left arm jutted out in an odd kind of salute.

"What was that?" I asked.

"I don't know. My arm just jerked." He didn't even interrupt the game. *Now what?* I wondered.

This type of seizure began to happen more often. Anything in his left hand was in danger, so we encouraged him to hold things in his right hand.

Each day brought a new crisis.

*Crash!*

It only takes a few seconds to run to any room from the furthest corner of the trailer, but in those few seconds my imagination ran riot. I knew the crash must be a dish of some sort. That gave me a clue where to run. On the kitchen floor a dinner plate lay shattered in a thousand pieces. I barely noticed it. I saw Jesse's head and shoulders on the kitchen table, his body still upright and in convulsions. It seemed an impossible position.

I said, as I had so many times before, "It's okay, honey. You're going to be okay." There was less panic in my voice now. I carried his stiff little body to the living room and put him down gently, keeping one eye on him and the other on the second hand of my watch. Once the convulsions abated I put him on the couch with a pillow and covered him with a blanket. I wiped the smudges of blood off the kitchen floor and walked to the bathroom to remove the splinters of glass from my foot.

The next day there was a call from a neighbour. Her kids had seen Jesse moving like a robot. Then he went down on his hands and knees. They thought he was looking at something under the trailer. The next time they looked, he was sleeping. I ran again. He was in a post-seizure sleep in the mud. I picked him up and carried him home.

Some days I let him walk to school. I was nervous about it, but I knew I had to give him some independence. Walking to school was on the "dangerous," but not the "most dangerous" list. It was harder for me to let him go alone than to drive him, and some days I worked myself into such a frenzy that I had to drive him for my own peace of mind. If his seizures were short and infrequent one week, I'd relax a bit and let him go, but it was usually when I relaxed enough to let my guard down that something went wrong.

On April 13th, he had gone six days without a seizure. There was only a half-day of school, so I decided to let him walk home at noon. Even so, Tara and I went out to meet him. We walked all the way to school without seeing a sign of him. We walked much faster on the way back. I carried Tara part of the way so she wouldn't slow me down. As we turned the corner and started the last block home, I spotted something in the ditch. It was Jesse, sleeping as soundly as if he was at home in bed.

Now when Jesse had a few days seizure-free, I insisted on driving him to school and picking him up afterwards. I was never at ease. When the seizures were frequent, I was afraid they would never end. When they were less frequent, I was afraid of what might come. It was almost impossible to hope any more. I tried to conceal my constant anxiety, but I'm sure Jesse saw through me. When I asked him about an episode at school one day, he assured me it was "just a little seizure."

At our next meeting, Dr. Lowry suggested we get the MRI scan done at either Montreal or Winnipeg. The Hospital For Sick Children in Toronto was another possibility. That decision he left up to us. Wherever we chose to go, they would do all the testing necessary to determine if Jesse might be a candidate for surgery.

By that time, Chris and I had almost accepted the idea of surgery. If the MRI showed that the seizures were caused by scarring, we would certainly consider it. Whatever it took to get rid of the seizures, we were determined to do.

It was at this meeting that Dr. Lowry confessed that Jesse's was the most difficult case he had ever encountered. Finally, it had been said: Jesse was not an average child with epilepsy. Our life was not the norm for families of a child with epilepsy. It was different, and because it was different, I was determined to get to the bottom of it.

Chris and I discussed the possibilities. Dr. Lowry had told us there was a neurological hospital in Montreal, and he agreed to speak to a neurologist there, a Dr. Andermann, about Jesse. In the meantime, I wrote to the Hospital for Sick Children in Toronto and asked their opinion on which hospital had the most experience with epilepsy surgery, frontal lobe epilepsy in particular.

*Reply from the Hospital for Sick Children, April 6th, 1988*

We have become more and more convinced based on our personal experience, surgery can be a major benefit to many children.

The Montreal Neurological Institute has had probably the world's largest experience when it comes to epilepsy surgery, but only a small proportion of the patients operated upon there are in the pædiatric age group. In fact, there would be few centres that have a large experience in pædiatric epilepsy surgery, and perhaps our own hospital has the most experience in Canada and perhaps North America. Most of these surgeries at all institutions are of the temporal lobe, so the number of children who have had frontal lobe epilepsy surgery would be small in all centres.

I think it is worthwhile for Jesse to be evaluated for epilepsy surgery, and this could be done well either in Montreal or here, and you would not be making a mistake with either choice.

A few days later, Dr. Lowry called with the news that he had spoken to the neurologist in Montreal and had sent Jesse's EEGs and CT scans down to him. Dr. Andermann would try to admit Jesse into hospital in Montreal in two or three months for an evaluation.

When the sky is falling, just looking for things to hold it up keeps you going. The worst that could come from this evaluation would be nothing, so we had nothing to lose. And possibly everything to gain.

Meanwhile, Jesse continued to have seizures, stomach-aches, and twitches, and his left arm periodically jerked out in that parody of a salute I had first seen when we were playing cards.

At the end of April I called the neurologist in Montreal and asked his secretary if she had heard anything about an admission date for Jesse. Dr. Lowry, she told me, should call Dr. Andermann the following Tuesday. I called the Hospital for Sick Children in Toronto and inquired about the waiting list for neurological evaluations.

On the Tuesday, Dr. Andermann informed Dr. Lowry that he would put Jesse on the emergency list and try to get him in some time in May. Toronto called back to say they were admitting for mid-July. It was a difference of two months: two more months of seizures, two more months of uncertainty and fear. We chose to go to Montreal.

On May 16th Jesse had another *grande mal* seizure. It proved to be another turning point. The children were on the floor in the living room, watching cartoons. Tara shouted that Jesse was having a seizure. As always, I ran to him. He was still convulsing. As I alternately looked at my watch and at him, I could see that this one seemed different. His head was jerking, but he was looking at me as if he could see me. I asked him if he was all right, and he *seemed* to say "yes." He didn't actually say the word. It was more a nod, or a look in his eyes, but he was definitely giving me some kind of confirmation. When the convulsions ceased, he jumped up and started playing. He began turning in circles.

"Look, Mom," he said as he swung his body around. Like a prop pinned to his shoulder, his left arm hung and swung freely. He then jerked his hip to the left. His arm and hand flew into the air and came down again with a sharp smack on his left side.

"Jesse, what are you doing?" I demanded. "What's wrong with your arm?

"I can't move it."

"Come here!"

He walked over to me, and I reached for his left arm. It felt cold, and lifeless as rubber. His right arm was fine, but his left arm was dead. He said he could feel me touching it, but he couldn't move the arm or his fingers. He wasn't scared. Slowly, the movement came back, to the arm first, and then the fingers. "It's okay now," he said, and went back to watching TV.

I was stunned. First the seizures scrambled his mind, then they changed his personality. Were they now going to cut off his limbs, one at a time? What would happen next time? Would he be paralysed from the neck down? Would it affect him for a few minutes at first, but eventually be permanent?

Three days later Jesse had another *grande mal*. He went into an absence seizure while he was eating breakfast. He began staring blankly, as usual, and turned his head to the left. He stared at Chris as though he could hear what his father was saying but couldn't answer. He stared with his mouth open and a silly smile on his face for the next few minutes. Then his head went back and to the left, and he blinked his eyes. Chris carried him to the couch as the rhythmic jerking began.

I was on the phone immediately. While I waited impatiently for our family doctor to come to the phone, I yelled at Tara to get on her bike and go to Bev's: "We'll have to take Jesse to the hospital!" The seizure had been going on for almost five minutes, but the doctor had not yet picked up the phone when they began to slow down. Then they stopped.

I looked out the window and saw my five-year-old daughter, panic stricken, peddling her two-wheeler as fast as she could go. I threw open the patio door. "Tara, come back," I called to her. "Jesse's okay now!"

She wheeled her bike around and came back home.

Tara, although only five and a half years old, handled things very well. Perhaps it was because she had experienced her own share of physical problems. She was born with her left eye slightly turned in. I didn't notice it much. After all, she was my beautiful baby girl. Other people noticed it more. I took her to an ophthalmologist when she was a few months old. He said it was just a lazy eye and to bring her back in a year or so. If it got worse, they could perform cosmetic surgery. "Nothing to worry about," he said, and I didn't think about it again for some time.

When she was two and we were living in Vanscoy, the problem seemed to be getting worse. This time an ophthalmologist in Saskatoon told us that her vision was very poor in that eye, and had been from birth. He prescribed glasses—one lens clear, the other as thick as the bottom of a Coke bottle. We were to put a patch over her good eye for a few hours each day so that she would be forced to use, and thus strengthen, her bad left eye. We did this for over a year, at which time she was scheduled for an operation which would tighten the outside muscle and make the eye look straight.

She was brought back to her room shortly after she had gone down for surgery. Her eye wasn't patched. Nothing had been done. The surgeon told us that, when he was ready to begin, he had noticed that the retina was partially detached. We would have to go to the Calgary Foothills Hospital to see a specialist. Meanwhile, we were to keep her as still as possible so the retina did not detach totally.

A few days later the arrangements had been made, and we drove to Calgary, where the specialist informed us—bluntly, and rather impatiently—that Tara did not need corrective surgery. She had a folded retina, not a detached one. There was nothing that could be done. She would never see anything but shadows through her left eye. We were to be cautious about keeping her good eye from harm. We were to go ahead with the cosmetic surgery to correct the inward turn, but we were to get rid of the glasses. They were not doing her any good, and never would.

This was our first experience with the detached, arrogant manner of some specialists. It would not be our last.

After Jesse's seizures began, Tara was understandably frightened at what was happening to her big brother. She cried once in a while, but she soon came to accept that this was the situation, and we—and she—would just have to deal with it. "It's not anyone's fault Jesse got sick," I told her. "I know it hurts, and I know it's hard, but we have to keep trying, and keep looking for answers."

The bond between Jesse and Tara was always strong. Once, when Tara was having a bout with tonsillitis, Jesse sat on the couch with her, holding her head in his lap. As he was nursing her and comforting her, he had a small seizure. The image is forever imprinted on my mind: the sick comforting the sick, with the open-hearted love and compassion of children.

*Diary entry, May 22nd, 1988*

Jesse had a seizure about 11:15 AM. I saw him coming out of it only. He hadn't looked good all day. He slept till 2:00. When he woke up, he had another seizure about ten minutes later. He stared for about two–three minutes, then he came out of it. He went to lay down again and fell asleep immediately for about ten more minutes. He got up and began eating again and had another seizure. This one lasted for one minute. He was able to answer "yes and no," slowly. But you could see he was in a seizure. Then he came out of it.

I called the hospital and after a huge run-around, I left my number with a resident neurologist. They told me Dr. Lowry was in Cincinnati, Ohio at meetings. Nevertheless, about fifteen minutes later Dr. Lowry called me and told me to bring Jesse to the hospital two days from now. He said he would check him at 8:30 AM and get a blood level done. He said the only thing they could do if he had any more problems is to admit him to hospital, and basically watch him.

I hope Montreal will call this week. They said "May," and this is the last week of May. We have to get something done. I am starting to go crazy.

We went in to have the blood test and to see Dr. Lowry at the appointed time. He gave Jesse a quick check-up, but there was nothing to see. As he wrote in his letter to Dr. Andermann in Montreal, "his intelligence is normal and his neurological examination is normal also."

"Dr. Lowry, he's having seizures in his sleep," I said. "The change to Depakene hasn't made any difference. He's getting worse"

"Maybe we should try another medication."

"I don't think it's a good idea right now. None of them seems to make any difference."

*He's running out of answers, too,* I thought.

"If Montreal doesn't call in a few days, maybe I could give them a call. But," he added, "there's not a whole lot I can do. It's not my hospital."

*There is a whole lot you can do,* I thought angrily. *If you put a little pressure on them, Jesse will get in sooner.*

Then he said, "You know, Mrs. Armstrong, I think of Jesse often. When I go home at night, many times I think of what I can do to help him. It's very frustrating for me, too, not being able to control his seizures."

This was the first glimmer I had that Chris and I were not the only ones lying awake wondering how to save Jesse.

*Diary entry, June 2nd, 1988*

Jesse said he wasn't feeling good. Said he had a stomach ache at about 8:00 AM. He had a seizure, but he still answered me and walked. He said he wanted to lie down. I knew he was in some kind of a seizure because his eyes were far away and glassy again. I put him in my bed and he slept right away. I woke him up at 8:40 for his medicine and he got up then.

His behaviour is still very bad. He doesn't care much about anything or anyone.

I called Dr. Lowry last Friday and left a message for him to call Montreal in the morning and get back to me. He didn't call Montreal or me. I called back at 4:00 and he simply said he thought it would be better if I called them again myself.

Chris called on Tuesday and the secretary said we were at the top of the list and it could be any day now. It may even be today. She said Dr. Andermann was inEurope now till July, but Jesse would be admitted under someone else for the testing. She said she would check into it. Today is Friday and they still haven't called.

I'm sick and tired of getting put off by everyone. If it was any one of their children, they would have been in there a long, long time ago. This is getting to be real bullshit.

I don't even know Jesse any more. I feel soon it will be too late. There'll be no turning back and I will never ever find my boy again.

Dr. Lowry called the next day to see how I had made out with Montreal. Two days later Jesse had more seizures in his sleep. Now he didn't even wake up when he went into convulsions. The following day he had three seizures in school. He slept after each one. After the third, his teacher called me to take him home. I brought him home and he had a few more, sleeping after each one. He woke up with a terrible headache after the last. I kept him on the couch with a cold cloth on his forehead.

I needed some direction, some reason to go on. I needed more faith. I prayed to God daily. I told him I would wait for an answer. I also prayed for guidance, and for strength while I waited.

I had been praying and reading the Bible frequently. I was distressed about my role in Jesse's life. If his destiny was predetermined, would my interventions have any effect? Shouldn't I just trust in God and wait for his plans to be realized?

I spoke to Jeanne, my oldest sister, whose husband had died twelve years earlier, leaving her with four small children. She had become close to God over the years. She explained to me what she saw and believed to be the truth. The forks and turns we choose to reach our destination are in our hands, she said, and how we get there is up to us. God gives us the tools to travel by. He gives us the wisdom to weigh the factors involved, the heart for a compassionate choice, and the courage and strength finally to choose the best course. He could create miracles independent of our actions, or he could work through science and medicine. In Jesse's case, Jeanne said, it looked like God was taking the long way around.

It looked that way to me, too.

I called Chris at work and asked him to call Dr. Lowry. I couldn't deal with the man again today. He left a message, and Dr. Lowry got back to him later. Chris told him Jesse was in bad shape. Dr. Lowry said we could increase his medication if he was having problems, but he was already on quite a high dosage and there wasn't much room to expand. Chris called Montreal again. The secretary was polite, but she couldn't give us any new information.

I called Montreal back on June 9th. I spoke to someone in admitting who told me they had a date set for June 29th. At last! I didn't know what was going to happen in Montreal, but I knew something was going to change. It had to. A person couldn't go on living like this.

I had three weeks to prepare for the trip. I phoned Saskatchewan Health and spoke to someone handling out-of-province applications. Dr. Lowry's office had already contacted them and they had done the preliminary paper work. Doris, Dr. Lowry's nurse co-ordinator, suggested that we apply to the Kinsmen Foundation for financial help. She arranged to send a letter from Dr. Lowry to the Foundation, describing Jesse's medical condition and the reasons for the consultation in Montreal.

The Kinsmen Foundation was wonderful. They approved our application and offered to pay for my air fare, meals, and lodging. Like many others, we had been living from pay cheque to pay cheque, and had no savings. We greatly appreciated the Kinsmen's generosity. They never once made us feel we were a charity case. Rather, they gave the impression that they felt blessed they could help.

Dr. Andermann's office recommended a rooming house two blocks from the hospital. I made a reservation for two weeks. I called the travel agent designated by the Kinsmen Foundation and arranged for departure on June 28th. The return flight was left open.

Chris would stay behind and continue to work—the bills still had to be paid—and Tara would stay at each of my sisters's homes for a few days at a time while I was away. No one was allowed any self-pity. "That's the way it is, and we just have to deal with it," was something I said often. Jesse was the only one I allowed to feel sorry for himself, and he chose not to.

Chris drove us to the airport. We stood at the Air Canada counter with our tickets in hand. The attendant spoke to Jesse with a warm smile. "Is this your first time on an airplane?"

"Yes," he said.

"Are you going for a visit?" she asked.

"No" he said. "They're going to fix my brain."

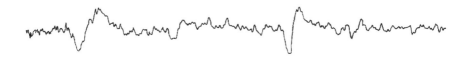

# 5 / The Montreal Neurological Institute

When the plane landed in Montreal I silently thanked God Jesse hadn't had a seizure on the flight. I asked Him to hold off a little longer. We found the baggage terminal by following the flow of traffic. It felt odd to have landed in a strange city with no one to meet us, but as soon as I heard the cab driver's accent I felt a sense of belonging and comfort. It was as if my Dad had sent one of his cousins to meet the plane.

The rooming house where we stayed was run by the elderly widow of a doctor who had worked at the Montreal Neurological Institute. She had a warm smile for Jesse, and asked all about him before showing us to our room. There she wished us a good night. It was June 28th, the eve of my thirty-first birthday.

The next morning, Jesse and I walked hand-in-hand up to the Institute. Built in 1934, it stands across the street from the Royal Victoria Hospital, to which it is connected by a third-floor walkway. From a distance the two buildings on the eastern slope of Mount Royal, with their stone exteriors and vine-covered walls, look like fairy-tale castles.

After Jesse was admitted, we were taken to the second floor and settled into a semi-private room. The window, with its dark wood casing around a twenty-four inch pane, looked out onto the wall of the adjacent building and a temporary parking lot for construction workers. We unpacked Jesse's suitcase and tried to make ourselves comfortable.

The hospital regulations were not drawn up with an active seven-year-old in mind. For starters, Jesse was not to walk around the room unescorted. When I wasn't with him, he was to remain in bed with the side rails up. I intended to be with him most of the time, anyway. At meal times I'd set up his tray and get him ready to eat with the television in front of him and the side rails up. Then I'd go across to the cafeteria in the Royal

Vic for my own meal, stopping for a quick smoke in the third-floor lounge on my way back.

Jesse was also supposed to use a wheelchair whenever he left the room. It soon became apparent that he and I would both go insane if his feet were never allowed to touch the floor. So between meals we would play Uno or take a deck of cards to the third-floor lounge. The nurses were too busy to be much concerned with where we went, as long as Jesse wasn't alone.

It was in the lounge that we met Ed. Most of the patients were from the surrounding area and spoke French. Many were bilingual, but some had no English at all. A few were from the United States. Ed's first language was English, but he was fluent in French, which he had learned as an adult. He was learning to walk again after having had a tumour removed from his leg. He was always willing to talk, and often came to visit Jesse. Sometimes the three of us would have a serious game of Uno. Other times, Jesse and I would teach Ed a new card game. We planned our games around Jesse's tests and Ed's therapy. Jesse was delighted to have someone to visit with other than me, and he enjoyed Ed's visits immensely.

Jesse was the only child in the hospital, but he was far from being the only patient awaiting epilepsy surgery. There were other patients with tumours, strokes, and head injuries. Most were there for an extended stay: weeks, even months on the ward was not uncommon. They each had a different story, each as tragic as the next. They spoke freely about seizures, head injuries, telemetry, and brain surgery, and every day someone had a story to tell about something that had happened on their ward that day.

It was common to see people walk into the lounge with their heads wrapped in bandages. Some would come in wheelchairs holding onto the metal boxes that contained all the connections to the EEG electrodes that were still glued to their scalp. They looked like creatures from a science fiction movie. I listened to some of their stories with amazement, doubt, incredulity; I found it unsettling that they should share these things so freely.

Each evening, when I returned to the rooming house, the landlady came to the door to ask about my day. I suspected she was lonely, and she loved to talk. She told me about her husband, whom she missed dearly, and showed me his room. She had kept it exactly as it had been the day he died, right down to his clothes laid across the freshly made bed. It gave me a chill, but it seemed to give her comfort.

By the first week-end, no testing had been done. On Saturday, Jesse had a *grande mal*. Sunday evening we acquired a room-mate, thirteen-year-old Jaime and her mother, Ivy, from Sault Ste. Marie. Jaime had a severe seizure disorder, the result of meningitis as a newborn. When she was awake and had the energy to talk, she was congenial, and had a delightful sense of humour. Ivy was very pleasant, although there was a part of her that seemed to have hardened. She had been through several lifetimes of pain in Jaime's thirteen years.

On Monday, July 4th, we finally met Dr. Andermann. He walked briskly into Jesse's room, his entourage three paces behind him, and stretched out a hand. "Hello, Mrs. Armstrong."

As I took his hand he continued, "Did you have a good trip?"

"Yes," I began. "We—"

"Good." The social amenities over, he proceeded to tell me about Jesse's proposed treatment: "The first step is to determine the cause of the hypodense area on his CT scan. It could be a tumour, a blood vessel, or scar tissue. When this is discovered, we move on to find out exactly where in the brain his seizures are originating, and how much area they are covering. Not all patients are surgical candidates. If he is operable, we will discuss it then."

"When do you expect to know?"

He peered at me over his glasses. "I can say nothing until the tests are completed. This will probably take a few weeks. You have a place to stay?"

"Yes, thank you. I—"

His right hand went up like a policeman stopping a lane of traffic. "Good." He turned around. The bank of residents parted to clear his path, and he strode away.

I came to know Dr. Andermann's stop-sign gesture very well. It meant, "End of conversation. Say no more. I am leaving now. Good-bye." If you paused after he answered a question, the stop sign went up. You had to think fast or the buzzer would go. *Too late, time's up.* I once blurted out another question after the stop-sign had gone up, and he was quite annoyed. I hadn't obeyed the signal. He answered quickly, then showed the stop sign again, turned, and walked away.

Dr. Andermann was Jaime's neurologist as well. Ivy had dealt with him before, and we joked about his brusque manner. If you weren't on the receiving end, it could be quite comical. In any case, rumour had it that he was an excellent neurologist.

The next day Jesse went down for an EEG. When the staff had heard they were getting a child, everyone wanted to be the technician on the test. It was a change for them, since the majority of their patients were adults. Francine won the draw. She was a short woman with dark hair and a positive outlook. She took an immediate liking to Jesse. As for Jesse, he adored her on sight.

She won me over when she told Jesse that he was being a good boy, although he was being nothing of the sort as she placed the electrodes on his head. She seemed to understand that Jesse wanted to please more than anything. Often he would ask, "Was I good today?" Sometimes he was. More often he was not, but I usually said, "Yes, Jesse, you were good," and a huge grin would spread across his face. Sometimes, though, I couldn't let things go by, and I'd have to point out what he had done wrong. He always looked surprised and disappointed. The fact was, he was progressively losing his social skills. He was unable to see the consequences of his actions. He saw it, he wanted it, he did it.

Now I sat with him as he lay on the bed with his head covered with wires. The perfect scenario would be for him to have a seizure while on the EEG so the machine could record it and discover its origin. Francine tried to provoke a seizure by having him open and close his eyes. When that didn't work, she suggested deep breathing. Still nothing happened. Then she had him watch a set of flashing lights. As a last resort, I started deep breathing with him, exaggerating each breath, urging him to continue. It was a long process, and it didn't seem to be getting us anywhere.

Suddenly Jesse looked to the left. I stood up and held his hands. His head slowly turned. His left eye and the left side of his mouth began to twitch. Then the convulsions started. Francine stayed at the machine, but immediately called in her colleagues. I was asked to move aside while they held Jesse down so that his violent movements would not break the connections of the electrodes on his skull.

The convulsions lasted about a minute and a half. Afterward, Jesse was dazed and tried to get up. I could tell that his left arm and hand were paralysed. The technicians talked to him and continued to hold him down so he wouldn't pull out the wires. He struggled for a few moments, then lay back and fell asleep.

Francine came in to me, letting the EEG run. "You did great," she said. "Now we'll record him sleeping for about twenty minutes."

Later that afternoon I questioned Dr. Curran, the resident who had admitted Jesse, about the EEG. He told me he was pleased that we'd been able to record a seizure. "But," he cautioned, "more tests have to be done, and we won't be able to come to any conclusions for some time."

In the next few days, Jesse underwent a battery of tests, including the Weschler Intelligence Scale for Children, the Weschler Memory Scale, the Vineland Social Maturity Scale, the Wingfield Object Naming test, the Children's Word Fluency test, and a hand Dynamometer test. In spite of how much he had lost in the eighteen months he'd been sick, the overall results put him in the low-average range. There was no way of telling what intelligence score he had started with, but from the events I had recorded in his baby book—when he first walked, talked, spoke in sentences, learned self-help skills—together with the gross deterioration I described, they concluded that Jesse had begun with above-average intelligence.

In addition to the psychological tests, Jesse had blood tests, skull X-rays, another EEG, and an MRI scan. Because it was imperative he be still during the MRI, Jesse was given an injection to make him sleep. The test proved inconclusive, however, because of the constant myoclonus Jesse experienced even while sleeping.

By Friday, they had completed the tests. Dr. Andermann invited us to his Monday morning conference where the specialists would go over Jesse's case. Ivy had once been through a similar conference with Jaime, and she filled me in on what to expect: "It's intimidating at first to sit in front of twenty, thirty doctors shooting questions at you, but just relax and you'll do fine."

"Thanks Ivy," I said, "but I'm not nervous. The thing that frightens me more than the possibility of surgery is the possibility that they won't be able to do anything."

This was our last hope of saving Jesse. It had to work.

After leaving the hospital that evening, I walked to a nearby corner store and picked up a few groceries, including fresh fruit and a few cans of pop. As I walked home, I remembered that the landlady had told me there was only one small fridge in the hallway, and it had to be shared by the guests in all three rooms. To be fair to the others, I was to use only a corner of it. It sounded reasonable to me, but what with my preoccupation with Jesse and the results of the conference on Monday, I had bought nearly two bags of groceries. *Oh, well,* I thought, *I'll just put one can of pop in the fridge at a time and keep most of the fruit in my room.*

I opened the door to the rooming house with difficulty, as I had the groceries, my purse, and a suitcase of Jesse's dirty laundry that I intended to take to a laundromat the next day. The landlady met me, as usual, but her smile changed to a look of outrage as she saw my groceries.

"Hello," I said, tentatively.

"I told you not to buy a lot of groceries!" she shouted at me. "There isn't much fridge space! There are others living here, you know!"

"Yes, I know. I just thought—"

"I told you! I told you!" she kept shouting. "I know you. I know your type. I knew when you walked in that you'd cause trouble!"

I couldn't believe what was happening. The woman was beginning to scare me. Her face was contorted with rage and she continued to shout.

My bags were getting heavier. I just wanted to go to my room and put them down.

When I was finally able to get a word in, I told her that I intended to keep most of it in my room and would use only a small space in the fridge. She turned on her heel without a word and stomped away. I was shaking all over as I climbed the stairs. I had visions of her coming up to my room in the night, using her key to get in, and . . . do what? I wasn't sure, but I was scared.

I walked quietly downstairs, slipped out the door, and ran to a pay phone across the street to make a collect call home. It was good to hear Chris's voice.

"Get out of there tomorrow," he told me. "Find another place, pay her what you owe and get out."

"But I'm scared," I said. "She lost it completely, Chris. What if she . . . I don't know . . . what if she comes after me, or something?"

I didn't know what I was scared of, except that I was alone in a strange city and my temporary "home" was run by a woman who seemed to have lost her mind.

"She's not going to hurt you," Chris said, and it was his calm reassurance that eventually gave me the courage to go back to my room. Even so, I slept only fitfully, and I was relieved when morning dawned.

Ivy gave me the address of a rooming house run by Catholic sisters where she was staying. On Sunday, I moved in. Ivy and I were able to come and go together to the hospital each day. The only inconvenience was that it was a half-hour from the Institute, and I had to take a bus and transfer, then cover the last four steep blocks on foot.

Still, I was much happier there. We were allowed to smoke in our rooms, and there was a chapel on the main floor, a cafeteria in the basement, a comfortable visiting area off the main door, and a pay phone on each floor. There was also a security guard after 7:00 PM, so I didn't have to worry about crazed landladies attacking me in the night. It was less expensive, too; what I spent on bus fare I saved in rent.

Ivy and I kept a rigid schedule. We were up at 7:00 AM and at the hospital by 8:00. We stayed until Jaime and Jesse where settled for the night, usually 8:00 or 9:00 PM. Then we retraced our steps to the convent. We rarely deviated from this schedule, and having one another's company made it easier.

On Monday morning, Jesse and I waited in the hall outside the conference room. We made up games to play as we waited, and I skimmed over my diary from the past year and a half. When they called us in, I was ready.

They asked Jesse to walk across the room, heel to toe. They asked him to close his eyes and extend his arms in front of him. They asked questions, made observations, consulted amongst themselves. Finally, Dr. Andermann said, "Jesse, I have one last question."

Jesse looked at him expectantly.

"Have you ever been in jail?" Dr. Andermann asked very seriously.

Jesse responded timidly: "No."

He didn't understand it was a joke. It was so far removed from what I had seen of Dr. Andermann's character that I barely knew it myself until the whole room chuckled.

Then we were dismissed. A short time later, Dr. Andermann called me to a small waiting room by the nursing station. Dr. Curran and a tall, dark, pleasant-looking man were with him. Dr. Andermann introduced me to Dr. Olivier. He extended his hand and I took it. It was as warm as his smile.

"Dr. Olivier is a neurosurgeon here, and he has performed many epilepsy surgeries," Dr. Andermann informed me. "We have discussed Jesse and gone over his history. We are all in agreement."

Dr. Olivier had the negatives from all the scans taken since Jesse first became ill. He held one up. "There," he said, pointing. "In the right frontal lobe." He held up another scan, then another. "It doesn't seem to be increasing in size, and there's nothing to indicate that the damage extends beyond this area." He tapped the negative with his finger. "The electroencephalogram also confirms that this area is the origin of the seizures. We don't believe it's a tumour; it's likely scar tissue."

"We think Jesse is a good candidate for surgery," Dr. Andermann broke in, "and we recommend Dr. Olivier perform it. You can speak more with Dr. Olivier this afternoon."

I thanked them and went back to Jesse's room. I had told Ivy I was more afraid of what they couldn't do for Jesse than what they could. But now, faced with the realization that my Jesse was going to have brain surgery, I was petrified.

After lunch I walked down to the main floor and into Dr. Olivier's office. We talked for over an hour. He never rushed me. He never cut me off. He answered all my questions completely and honestly, telling me the mortality rate associated with this type of surgery as well as the success rate. He was human and compassionate, and by the end of our meeting I trusted him completely.

"Will Jesse be in pain after the surgery?" I asked.

"No. The brain doesn't feel pain. The incision will be sore. There will be swelling from the intrusion on the brain, which might be uncomfortable. He might have a headache. On the whole, however, there's not a lot of pain associated with brain surgery."

"When would you do it?" I asked.

"I'm leaving for holidays on Friday. I'll be gone four weeks. We could wait until I get back, or we could do it on Wednesday."

"Wednesday?" I repeated, stunned.

"Yes."

"You mean *this* Wednesday, the day after tomorrow?" I could hardly catch my breath. "Don't you need to do more testing?"

He shook his head. "I'm satisfied with the results we have."

Brain surgery some time in the future was hard enough to grasp. But *Wednesday?*

Dr. Olivier reassured me: "I want you to understand, Mrs. Armstrong, we don't go into surgery blindly. Your son has been well documented. The examinations have been thorough. I don't believe further testing will uncover anything new or change our decision. If you decide to proceed with surgery, then the only question is the timing. Delaying it will not change the outcome, but it will give you more time to think."

"Do you think Jesse's ready?" I asked.

"Jesse is ready," he replied, "but you and your husband must feel comfortable with the decision. I can only assure you that, from a surgical point of view, we will be just as prepared on Wednesday as we will be four weeks from now."

"I'll have to talk to Chris," I said. "I can't decide this on my own."

"Of course. We won't do anything until both you and your husband have had a chance to discuss it. Then if you still feel Wednesday is too soon, we can wait until later." He gave me his card. "If you have any further questions, don't hesitate to call me."

I rose slowly from my seat, worried I might have missed something. I couldn't possibly have asked all the questions I should have, but I couldn't think of any more. I walked quietly up the stairs to Jesse's room. Things had been happening so slowly up to this point. Now they were happening too fast.

Ivy offered to stay with Jesse while I phoned Chris. I reached him at work. I told him what Dr. Olivier had said. We talked it over. Eventually, despite our fears, we agreed that our acceptance and readiness would be no greater four weeks from now than they were now. If they were prepared to go ahead with surgery, so were we. I went back to Dr. Olivier's office and told him that Chris would be catching a flight tomorrow so he could be here for the surgery on Wednesday.

Jesse, when I told him, was neither frightened nor concerned. I suspect he thought of surgery as just another test they had to do. I had never gone into it in detail with him. Plenty of time for that later, I'd thought.

"The doctors have looked at all your tests," I told him, speaking slowly. "They think you should have surgery."

"Okay."

"They'll put you to sleep on Wednesday, and Dr. Olivier will do the operation to try to get rid of your seizures. Dad's coming tomorrow, so he can be with us when you have the operation."

"When's he going to get here?"

"I'm not sure. Probably late tomorrow afternoon, or after supper."

"All right! Is Tara coming?"

"No."

"I miss her."

"I know, Jesse, but it's a long trip, and we'll go home soon, okay?"

"Okay," he said. "Do I have to have another EEG?"

"Not before the surgery, but probably some time after. They'll have to shave your hair, but it'll grow back. You'll look like a punk rocker."

"All right!"

"When you wake up, you might have a headache. Your head will be in bandages. Dad and I will be there. Are there any questions you want to ask me?"

"Do you want a game of cards?"

"Sure," I said. But I didn't want to play cards. I just wanted to hold him until Wednesday.

Bev called that night. She said they would be praying for us, and if there was anything she could do or anything I wanted, I was to call her. But I knew that already.

My sisters called. So did a friend from Calgary. They were all praying for a successful operation. I needed to hear that.

When Chris arrived, Jesse was delighted. He proudly introduced his Dad to Ed, Ivy, Jaime, and all the nurses. We played cards with Jesse for most of the day, and stayed with him until he fell asleep that night. We had taken a room at a bed-and-breakfast hotel not far from the hospital. Neither of us slept much.

Jesse's surgery was scheduled for 8:30. We were at the hospital by 6:30. After the IV was set up, Dr. Olivier and two residents, Dr. Smith and Dr. Farmer, came to speak with us.

"The operation will take about six hours," Dr. Olivier said. "I'll speak with you as soon as it's over. It will be a long wait, but try not to worry. We'll take good care of him."

We shook hands, and he went to the Operating Room to prepare while the two residents transferred Jesse onto a gurney. They wheeled him out the door. Chris and I walked beside the gurney.

"Can we go with him to the OR?" I asked.

"No," Dr. Smith said brusquely, at the same time Dr. Farmer said, "Oh, yes." Dr. Smith pursed his lips, but Dr. Farmer ignored him. "You can come as far as the doors."

They stopped the gurney in front of the double doors, then stepped back to let us say good-bye to Jesse.

"Remember Jesse, when you wake up Mom and Dad will be right there with you." I was determined to keep my voice steady. "I love you, honey-bear. Everything's going to be okay."

"Love you, son," Chris echoed.

They wheeled him through the doors, and he was gone.

I felt an urge to run after them. *Hold that knife, put down the mask, withdraw that needle! There will be no surgery today on my honey-bear! I've changed my mind!* Instead, Chris and I stared at the doors for a few seconds, then he reached for my hand and we walked away.

The next hours were the longest we had ever experienced. We went to the third-floor lounge and spoke with Ed and the other regulars. Nothing any-one said seemed to be of any significance. We watched the clock. I tried not to think about what they were doing to our son. We went to the chapel and said a prayer. We went for lunch. Neither of us ate. We played cards. Then it hit me again: *This is real. They're performing brain surgery on Jesse. How did it come to this? How could we allow it?* I had to make a conscious effort to pull myself back from the edge of hysteria.

At 2:00 o'clock we went to Jesse's room, waited half an hour. Back to the lounge for a smoke, then back down. At 3:00 I went up again, alone this time. Five minutes later I came back down. From the stairwell, I could see into Jesse's room. Dr. Olivier was speaking to Chris. I ran down the stairs and burst through the doors. "How is he?"

"He's doing fine. The operation went well. He's in ICU now, where he'll be monitored for the next twenty-four hours."

*Thank you God, thank you, thank you.*

"We removed about one-third of his frontal lobe," Dr. Olivier went on. "The abnormal tissue seemed to extend somewhat beyond this point, but we couldn't go any further. The good news is, it definitely wasn't a tumour."

"Will his seizures be gone?"

"They should be diminished. As for complete cessation, only time will tell. He may have some seizures in the next forty-eight hours. Those aren't a complication of surgery, or an indication that the operation failed. They're simply a post-op reaction to the trauma to the brain. They're to be expected."

I barely took in his words. "Can we see him now?"

"Give ICU a few moments to get him settled. Someone will be along shortly to let you know when he's ready."

ICU called an hour later. I was afraid of what I would see, but my need to see him was stronger than my fear.

Jesse lay naked on a narrow bed, a thin sheet covering the lower half of his body. His face was swollen, his eyelids puffy, his face pale. His head was wrapped in white gauze. A drainage tube carried a trickle of reddish-pink liquid from the back of his head into a glass container. He was connected to a respirator, a heart monitor, a nasal gastric tube, and an IV. His pulse rate flashed and beeped rhythmically on a monitor above his head.

I bent over the tubes and connections and softly kissed him on the cheek. "Hi, Honey-bear. It's Mommy. Daddy's here, too. You're doing really well. The operation is over, and you're going to be okay. We love you so much, Jesse."

"Hi, Bud," Chris said. "You did very good, Jesse. Dad's real proud of you."

Jesse opened his eyes slightly, closed them again.

I touched his hand, careful not to disturb the IV needle. All of a sudden, his heart rate went up. The beeping grew louder and more continuous. I looked wide-eyed at Jesse, at the monitor, back to Jesse.

"What's happening?" I demanded.

Jesse opened his eyes, turned to the left, and started to convulse.

# 6 / Rasmussen's Syndrome

Two nurses came running. Chris and I backed away. In a minute it was over. I had been told to expect it, I know, but I'd hoped Jesse might be spared these post-operative seizures. He'd been through so much already.

"Please, I want to see Dr. Olivier," I told the nurse.

Dr. Olivier was not in the hospital. They sent Dr. Smith.

"Could you check him? He just had a *grande mal*."

"We told you to expect that," he said coldly.

"I need to know he's okay."

Dr. Smith walked to the head of the bed and called Jesse's name. Jesse didn't stir. He returned to the foot of the bed and dug his thumbnail into the base of one of Jesse's toenails. Still nothing. He dug harder. Jesse stirred. Clearly, he was in a deep sleep, but he was responding to the pain. *All right,* I thought. *I get your point.* But Dr. Smith wouldn't let up until Jesse started to whine and thrash about, trying to move his foot.

"What are you doing?" I was furious. "You're hurting him!"

"You have to wake him up somehow," he said flatly, then turned and walked out.

Chris's parents and his brother Shawn arrived late, driving down to Montreal from Richmond Hill. Mom and Dad Armstrong were exhausted and went straight to their hotel, but Shawn came up to the hospital that night. The three of us went into ICU whenever they would let us until about 10:00 PM.

Before we went to bed I called my sister Henriette and asked her to call the rest of the family. The surgery went well, I told her, but they didn't get all the epileptic tissue. "Time will tell," I said. I was exhausted, but glad the day was over and elated that Jesse was going to be all right.

At noon the following day, he was transferred back to his room. The respirator and nasal gastric tube had been removed, but he was still hooked up to the heart monitors and the IV. His left eye was swollen shut, and I couldn't help noticing the myoclonus. I didn't have to be touching him to feel it. I could see it.

Someone—often all five of us—was with Jesse throughout the day, until eventually Felicia, the head nurse, came in to tell us that Jesse could hear us, even though he appeared to be sleeping. She asked us to speak more quietly. Rest was vital to Jesse's recovery. I was embarrassed by her gentle admonishment, but I was glad of it, too. It reassured me that her first concern was for Jesse.

Dr. Olivier came by with the two residents, Dr. Farmer and Dr. Smith. He would be leaving tomorrow, he said, and the residents would be taking care of Jesse.

I asked Dr. Olivier if I could speak with him alone. The residents left. I was frank: "I will not have Dr. Smith touching Jesse again, and I won't deal with him. He's rude and he's cruel." I told him about his objecting to our going with Jesse to the OR, and about his attitude in the ICU. "The man has a rotten attitude," I concluded, "and I don't trust him."

Dr. Olivier wished I would reconsider. "Dr. Smith may not have a good bed-side manner, but I assure you he is very competent. Think it over. Give him a second chance."

Had it been anyone but Dr. Olivier, I would have refused.

All the tubes and monitors were removed the next day. Jesse began smiling and talking, and he started to eat. We were all pleased with his progress, and he was especially pleased when a nurse wrapped the head of his teddy bear with gauze bandages like his own.

That day, July 15th, was our tenth anniversary. Chris and I had supper away from the hospital, then went back to be with Jesse.

By the end of the following day the swelling had gone down. Chris's parents and his brother left for home. On Sunday we said good-bye to Chris, who had to return to work. If all went well, the doctors said, Jesse and I would be able to go home in a week.

All did go well, or so it seemed. Jesse continued to recover. His voice was distressingly flat and expressionless, but Dr. Curran assured me that was common after surgery, and would undoubtedly diminish with time. The myoclonus had diminished as well, though I still harboured a horrible fear that *it* was not gone. I hoped I was wrong. Indeed, all the evidence pointed to it. Jesse hadn't had a seizure since the one in the ICU.

We continued to meet with Ed for Uno or cards. I continued to go to the third-floor lounge to smoke and speak with the regulars. Ivy and I still rode the bus to and from the hospital. It was nice to have someone who understood what Jesse and I were going through. As Ed was going to be discharged on Thursday, we decided to go out for supper on Saturday night. Ivy and I made plans to pick him up after we left the hospital that evening.

On Wednesday, Dr. Smith came to remove Jesse's stitches. I remembered my promise to Dr. Olivier. *Okay*, I thought, *I'll give the jerk a second chance.* I smiled at him, and hoped it didn't look as artificial as it felt.

He removed the bandages in silence. When they were off, I asked, "How does the scar look to you? Does it look like it's healed well?"

"What does it look like to *you?*" he snapped.

"This is the first scalp incision I've seen," I snapped back. "I assumed you had some previous experience to compare it to."

He said nothing more. He removed the stitches in silence, then gave Jesse a J-cloth cap.

*So much for second chances,* I thought.

When I arrived at the hospital Friday morning, Jesse was still asleep. Something wasn't right. He'd been seizure-free for eight days. Had our luck run out? He woke up with a headache and wanted to stay in bed. Later he had an absence seizure, and fell asleep again. When he awoke he had another. I knew for certain, then, that *it* had returned. Rather, *it* had never left.

This was rock bottom. The child had been assaulted off and on by his own body, his own brain, for a year and a half. He'd been poked and prodded, tested and sliced. His mental capacities had diminished. His memory was deteriorating. He was becoming socially handicapped and physically uncoordinated. Now the surgery that was supposed to have corrected it all hadn't worked. Surely, nothing worse could happen.

At 12:00 noon something worse happened.

Dr. Andermann came in, with Dr. Curran and the rest of the entourage behind him. His voice was as toneless as Jesse's: "Mrs. Armstrong, would you come with us?"

I looked at Dr. Curran. He wasn't smiling. I looked at Ivy. She nodded, indicating that she would keep an eye on Jesse. I walked beside Dr. Andermann. Dr. Curran and the rest followed. I said, "Jesse had two absences this morning. He's been seizure-free for eight days."

No one said a word.

We walked into a small examining room. Dr. Andermann motioned for me to sit down. He sat in front of me. One of the residents took a seat. Dr. Curran remained standing. Someone shut the door. Dr. Andermann got right to the point: "We took a specimen of Jesse's brain during surgery, and did a biopsy. The results came up this morning. Jesse has a rare brain disease called Rasmussen's Encephalitis."

I stared at him in disbelief. I must have misunderstood. But everyone was silent. All eyes were on me. I sensed Dr. Curran positioning himself, ready to catch me should I fall. *Do I scream now?* I wondered. *Do I start crying?*

"What are you talking about?" I asked. "Jesse doesn't have a disease!"

Dr. Andermann was annoyed with me for contradicting him. "Rasmussen's Encephalitis, or Rasmussen's Syndrome, is an inflammation of the brain which seems to affect only children," he said. "The disease is almost always confined to one hemisphere—in Jesse's case, the right."

I couldn't believe what I was hearing. The room was getting smaller. It was becoming a miniature torture chamber. I looked at each of the doctors in turn, willing someone to tell me this wasn't so. They all avoided my gaze. Dr. Curran's eyes were filled with pity, but he, too, was silent.

I turned back to Dr. Andermann. "Okay," I said, trying to think while I was speaking. Something could be done. Whatever it was, we would do it. If we had to stay in Montreal another three weeks, another three months, we would do it. "What's available to him? What's the cure?"

"There is no cure."

"Wha – what's going to happen to him?" I stammered. I couldn't bear it if anything *more* happened to him.

"There are still many unanswered questions," he said. "We have seen forty-eight patients with this syndrome. The inflammation damages the cells in the affected hemisphere. The seizures progressively worsen, and there is continued deterioration."

I was crying now as I asked him, almost in a whisper, "Is he going to die?"

"It is extremely rare to die of the disease itself. What most often happens is that the deterioration continues until paralysis is established and the affected hemisphere is destroyed. We then remove the diseased hemisphere in the hope of arresting the seizures."

"Could you be wrong?" I was grasping at straws, but straws were all I had. "Could there be a mistake?"

"No, I don't think we made a mistake. We have diagnosed forty-eight cases of this disease without error. Dr. Robitaille, our pathologist, is extremely competent."

"How did he get this disease?"

"There is still very little known about the disease, including its etiology. I suggest you speak with your husband. . . ."

*God, no! I can't tell Chris!* He had once told me that he didn't know what he would do if something happened to Jesse. This was definitely *something*.

"Dr. Andermann," I pleaded, "I can't tell my husband alone. Will you speak to him with me? I won't know what to say. He'll have questions. I won't be able to answer them."

"When you call him, you can tell him to contact me and I'll speak with him." He began to rise from his chair.

"You don't understand!" I was panicking. "You have to help me tell him about this!"

He looked at me, nodded. "All right," he said.

We tried calling then and there. Chris was out.

"When you do reach him," said Dr. Andermann, "tell him that I will be available to speak to him." With that, he rose and left. The other doctors followed him out.

I sat there, tears streaming down my face. Now I knew what *it* was. The insidious, unscrupulous thief who had been robbing my son of his life for eighteen months finally had a name. Rasmussen's Encephalitis. We would come to know that name well.

Felicia walked by. I thought Dr. Andermann had sent her to comfort me, but her first question was, "What's wrong?"

"Don't you know?"

"No, what's the matter?"

"Jesse has a brain disease!" I blurted it out and began to cry again.

"Oh, I don't think so. What gives you that idea?"

"Dr. Andermann just told me. He said it was Rasmussen's something-or-other."

Her expression changed to shock, then sympathy. She whispered, "Rasmussen's Encephalitis?"

I nodded. "I need a smoke, please. I have to get myself together before I see Jesse."

There was no smoking in the Institute, but Felicia brought me a tuna can ashtray. She shut the door and stayed with me until I was calm enough to go back to Jesse.

An hour had gone by.

As I walked in, Ivy looked up. She knew something was wrong. Dr. Andermann didn't spend that much time with a patient's family just to chat. "What's wrong?"

I whispered, "They told me Jesse has a rare brain disease."

She hugged me, and I nearly dissolved into tears again. Then I thought of Jesse. He was watching me.

"No," I said, and I pushed Ivy away. I opened my eyes wide to hold back the tears, shook my head back, and took a deep breath. I whispered, "I have to be strong for Jesse. I'll talk to you about it later." Turning to Jesse, I said, "Have any seizures while I was gone?"

"Just one," he said.

"It was an absence, about a minute," Ivy said.

"Want a game of cards?" I asked.

*I'm not telling him. If he asks, I'll give it to him in bits, introduce the villain gradually. But I'm not going to tell him voluntarily.*

I was fairly certain he wouldn't ask. He'd been getting progressively poorer at judging expressions, and progressively less aware of and less interested in his surroundings. He just wanted to play and be happy.

"Sure," he said. He wasn't too chipper, though. The seizure had left him with a mild headache, and he had his "having-a-bad-day-with-seizures" look which I was to become all too familiar with.

After one game, I left to call Chris again. There was still no answer. I dreaded having to tell him, but I was increasingly anxious to get it over with.

Ed came in later. He and Ivy and I went out for a smoke, onto the balcony adjoining our floor. Ivy had been waiting for the news. Ed was unaware anything was wrong. I wasn't looking forward to repeating the things I'd been told. I'd only managed to get through the past few hours by willing myself to forget about it for the present. I would think about it later. Right now I had to get through the day at the hospital with Jesse.

I blinked, swallowed, and took a deep breath. I began slowly: "They got the biopsy back today. Jesse has a brain disease." The tears began to fall, slowly—only a crack in the dam. "They said his seizures will continue. They'll become more frequent, and his brain will deteriorate."

Ed was stunned. Ivy put a hand on my shoulder. I was rigid. I felt alone. Ed gave me a hug and mumbled something about being so sorry, having to leave, seeing us tomorrow. I finished my cigarette. "I have to get back to Jesse."

Jesse had two more seizures. I wondered if the day's total of five was a precursor of what was to come.

It was after nine by the time I got home. I went to the pay phone on my floor. I dialled our number. Chris picked up the phone. I took a deep breath. "Chris, I've got some bad news."

I could feel his tension two thousand miles away.

"They did a biopsy on some of the tissue they took out during surgery. . . ." I paused after each sentence to muster the courage to speak the next. "The biopsy came back today. They say Jesse has a rare brain disease. . . . It's called Rasmussen's Encephalitis."

Chris's voice was immediately filled with resentment and anger. I understood them both. "What are you talking about?" he demanded.

"Dr. Andermann told me today. I tried calling you all day, but I couldn't reach you."

I paused for a response. There was none.

"It's a kind of inflammation of one hemisphere of the brain," I continued.

Then Chris began to cry. This was breaking him apart. I scrambled for something to calm him.

"Chris, he's not going to die. It's going to be hard, but we'll get through it. And Jesse will be okay." I had to believe that.

"What's going to happen to him?" he asked in a whisper.

"This disease strikes only children. It affects one hemisphere of the brain. The seizures get progressively worse. Sometimes the inflammation burns itself out before it destroys thewhole hemisphere. Sometimes it goes through the whole hemisphere until it paralyses one side of the body. I don't know a lot about it. *They* don't know a lot about it. There's no cure. But it doesn't usually cross over to the other hemisphere."

There was no response.

"Chris, you have to call my sisters and get them to tell Mom. And you'll have to tell Bev and Faye. They need to know."

"I can't." His voice was very small. "You'll have to tell them."

"I'll call your parents in Toronto. But Honey, I can't phone everybody else. I have too much to deal with here. Please, we have to be strong for Jesse. It's going to be okay. We'll make it." I paused. "I'll speak with Dr. Curran tomorrow, and with Dr. Andermann on Monday. I'll call you when I know more. It's going to be okay."

Chris hung up without another word. I guess I was the pillar of strength that day. It wasn't like me, and it was a hard role to play.

I dialled the operator to make a collect call to Toronto, then went through it all again with Chris's mother. They were still just sounds coming out of my mouth. I couldn't let myself feel them too deeply, not yet.

She was concerned about Jesse, of course, but also about me, one mother to another. "Is there anything I can do?" she asked. "Would you like me to come to Montreal?"

"Thanks, Mom," I said. "There's nothing you can do here, but I appreciate the offer."

"You call me if you need anything," she said. "Anything at all."

I promised I would, and I promised I would keep her informed. Then I hung up. My head felt as though it was going to burst. I barely made it to my room. I shut the door, dropped my bags, and fell to my knees. The strength drained out of me. Over and over, I called out, *Oh God, my baby, my baby, Oh God, my baby!*

Every limb, every organ, every molecule of my body screamed for help. I pleaded for strength, and none came. Finally I pulled my body onto the bed and cried myself to sleep.

Throughout the night I woke up in the clothes I had worn all day, looked into the darkness, realized it wasn't a bad dream, and cried myself to sleep again.

# 7 / Experimental Treatment

That Saturday was the night we had arranged to go out for supper. Ivy and Ed asked if I wanted to cancel. I said we should go ahead; I didn't want to rain on everyone's parade. Despite my good intentions, my spirits dampened everyone else's, so we cut the evening short.

On Sunday I met with Dr. Curran. I learned that Rasmussen's Encephalitis (sometimes called Chronic Encephalitis) had been identified in 1958 by Theodore Rasmussen, working at the Montreal Neurological Institute. Dr. Curran gave me a paper Dr. Rasmussen had written in 1978. I asked to borrow a medical dictionary for the evening. For at that moment I resolved to become an expert on the subject. I was not going to be caught off guard again. From now on I would know what to expect.

That night I began to read the report. I circled each word I didn't recognize and put a number beside it. On the back of each page, I wrote the number of the word and the meaning I had found in the medical dictionary. It was like learning a new language:

Encephalitis: inflammation of the brain
Hemiparesis: weakness of one side of the body
CSF: cerebrospinal fluid
Atrophy: decrease in size, wasting

I studied into the early hours of the morning, and on Monday I again spoke with Dr. Andermann. He told me about a new theory which had been proposed at the recent International Symposium on Rasmussen's Encephalitis. The theory postulated that something had gone awry with the immune system, and that a trial of immunosuppression and steroid therapy might prove beneficial in terminating or decelerating the progress of the disease. Several patients in France had been on this trial for the past year, and the therapy looked promising. Coincidentally, Jesse was the first patient diagnosed with the condition following the conference.

"We feel your son would be a good candidate for Cortisone therapy," Dr. Andermann told me. "He's still in the very early stages of the illness. There is the potential for preserving a great deal, compared with most of the patients we have seen."

"Did you say Jesse is in the *early* stages of the illness?"

He nodded. "Your son's neurological exam is normal. His intelligence is low-average. His gait is normal, and there is no weakness of the left side of his body. His seizures, although difficult to control, are not extremely frequent. As the disease progresses, his intellectual capabilities will diminish further, the seizures will become much more frequent, and a hemiparesis will develop."

"But he's already lost so much." I must have been in shock. "How can this be the early stages?"

"It is a cruel illness with no cure, Mrs. Armstrong. That's why I believe a trial of immunosuppression is indicated, to see if we can delay its progress."

"What you're saying, then, is that there is no alternate therapy, and we've got nothing to lose."

"That's right."

"Except for the side-effects of the drugs."

"Over the short term, the side-effects are minimal. I will discuss the protocol with Dr. Antel, our neuro-immunologist. Your son's treatment will be similar to that of organ transplant patients."

Later that day, Dr. Antel examined Jesse and went over the basic functions of the immunosuppressants so I would have some information to pass on to my husband when I spoke with him. I called Chris that evening. He was still extremely distressed. I told him about the experimental treatment. At least now, I said, there was a possibility of a plan of therapy, a glimmer of hope. I told him I would find out more about the side-effects when I met with Dr. Antel again the next day. Then the final decision would rest with us.

I questioned Dr. Andermann again, but he simply reiterated his recommendation. Without this experimental treatment, all we had to look forward to was the accelerating destruction of our child.

"We would like to keep you in Montreal at least two weeks from the time we start the drugs," he told me, "in order to monitor Jesse. Once you get back to Saskatchewan, he will have to continue being monitored as an out-patient. Weekly blood tests will be necessary. We will undertake to educate Dr. Lowry on the disease and the procedures he will have to follow."

On Thursday, July 28th, I saw Dr. Antel again. He and Dr. Andermann had developed a protocol: "The program consists of three drugs, Cyclosporin, Imuran, and Prednisone. With short-term use, there should be no serious, lasting side effects. We would like to put Jesse on a trial of a year, which I consider to be short-term. Because these are medications which alter the immune system, Jesse's red and white blood cell count may decrease and he may be susceptible to infections. Also, there may be a weight gain from the Prednisone, which is a steroid. We will be monitoring him closely."

I spoke to Chris again that night. He didn't seem quite as panicked as he had the night before. We decided to go ahead with the treatment. It seemed we had no other choice.

On Friday, I was introduced to Susan and her daughter Jill. They were in for Jill's one-year check-up following a hemispherectomy. She had been stricken only three months before half her brain was destroyed and had to be surgically removed. I inspected Jill carefully, watching her every move. I wondered if she was the same child inside that her parents had known before *it* had come to their house. I wondered if they had had time to notice the change and mourn the loss.

Jill was a pretty girl, and extremely active. Her limp was pronounced, though, and her left arm hung motionless at her side. She spoke well and seemed bright. I asked Susan about the whole experience—the deterioration, the operation, the recovery. She said the disease had progressed so quickly it was like a blur, and she hadn't had time to think about it. Our thieves were the same, then, but their MOs were different. Even so, I now had a better image of the disease. It lifted my spirits because it took away some of my fears and broke through my ignorance. Jill wasn't just a textbook case; she was a concrete example of what life after Rasmussen's could be.

Week-ends were the most difficult times. It was then that I missed Tara and Chris the most. The hospital was virtually deserted. There were few visitors, and the doctors were at a minimum.

Many patients were in for extended periods, and the number of visitors they received tended to dwindle with time. You could always recognize a newcomer by the amount of company he had. Other patients, like us, had come long distances to be treated at the institute, and had no relatives or friends living nearby.

A woman named Sarah was in the room next to ours. Her husband, Martin, came every day, as he had done for the past ten years. During a simple operation a decade earlier, there had been unexpected complications, and Sarah was left unable to speak, walk, or understand speech. She sat in a wheelchair in the hall, her head down, a tube running out of her nose. She was thin and frail, and she looked much older than she was. Her only means of communication was to utter a shrill scream, or to moan continuously. The sound sent chills up my spine. At first I felt sorry for the woman, but before long I wondered if we wouldn't go crazy with this moaning and screaming going on day and night. Nevertheless, it wasn't long after when it became just another sound on the ward.

On Saturday, Ivy and I obtained day passes and decided to "blow the joint" for a few hours. Jesse had been in the hospital for over a month now, Jaime nearly as long. It was a beautiful summer day. With the children secure in wheelchairs, we headed for the door. The summer air was an unbelievable lift to the spirits. We kept a firm grip on the wheelchairs as we raced down the steep hill.

"Wheee! Wheee!" we shouted. "We're free!"

There was a small playground two blocks away. We parked the chairs and let our passengers out. We were there for a few minutes when Jesse grabbed his stomach and began to stare. Two minutes . . . three minutes. . . . I began to worry. *Please let him come out of it.* Four minutes. He began to relax and fall asleep. I put him gently back in the wheelchair and we all walked back up the steep hill.

Jesse had six more seizures that day. He slept after each one, drained of colour and strength. By evening I insisted someone be called to examine him. A resident was sent.

"Jesse's had eight seizures so far today," I told him. "He really doesn't feel well. Isn't there something you can do?"

"I can give him an Ativan. It's a sedative, much like Valium. But you must realize that this is part of the progression of the Encephalitis."

*No, I don't have to realize that,* I thought. *All we need to know is that he's not feeling well. He hasn't been feeling well all day. Eight seizures is enough, thank you, whatever the cause. Just because we know what's responsible for them now doesn't mean he can tolerate them any better, or that it hurts me any less to see him this way.*

The next morning Jesse had another seizure. He fell asleep, only to wake up to another. I watched him as he turned to the left and stared blankly. I held his hands as usual and told him it was going to be okay. Suddenly his face turned blotchy, pure white with rosy stains. I pressed the buzzer for a nurse, but as she arrived his colour returned and the seizure ended. But now I had another category of seizure to add to the list.

After the fourth seizure in the morning he was given an Ativan. It put him to sleep for most of the day, but at least the seizures stopped. I didn't like the idea of sedating him. But with this disease, it seemed, you were always choosing the lesser of two evils.

By Monday, I felt as drained as Jesse. If I was afraid for his life now, I was terrified for his future. I was weak with worry when I ran into Dr. Curran in the hall.

"I don't think I can go on," I told him. "I can't manage this. I don't know what to do." I searched his eyes, looking for an answer, anything. *Just help me.*

"You're doing fine," he said. "You're strong, and you'll get through this. We'll begin the immunosuppression trial tomorrow. This may be the answer. Have hope."

I had an abundance of hope. It was faith I needed.

The program began the next day. Jesse was put on Imuran, Prednisone, and Cyclosporin in addition to Depakene and Tegretol. Dr. Curran gave me some papers on the new drugs. Again I borrowed the medical dictionary and went back to the rooming house to study.

Ivy and Jaime were leaving on Saturday. I was going to miss them. I wasn't looking forward to being alone again. Ed still came to visit regularly, and I continued to chat with the other patients. Only a few of them had been there as long as we had.

Norman was one of them. He looked to be twenty-five or thirty years old. He had been in a car accident and suffered from amnesia. His short-term memory was also poor. He spoke very little English. I could understand some French, but spoke only a little. Our conversations were meagre. A smile, a nod. "Hello, how are you today?" Norman could never remember the way back to his ward, so when he was ready to leave the smoking lounge, he would ask one of us to walk him back.

One day a visitor interpreted for us. I asked Norman how long he had been in the Institute. Norman shrugged, indicating that he wasn't sure. Our interpreter whispered to me, "Seven years." Norman heard, and was shocked. "Bien non! C'est vrais? Sept ans?"

I felt awful. I had anticipated neither the answer nor Norman's reaction. I could only hope that he would forget this conversation, too.

There were many sad situations. So many people had been robbed from inside. But there were miracles, too. There was a teenaged boy who had been in a car accident. I first saw him in the lounge with his parents. He was paralysed below the neck, and would often slip down in his wheelchair. His parents pulled him up again, but he always slipped back down. His eyes were vacant. He drooled continually. When they spoke, he didn't respond. But each week there was some improvement, until at last he was able to put his hand around a cup and drink through a straw. Then life returned to his eyes. He began to carry on conversations with his parents. He no longer drooled or slipped in his chair. We knew he would make it.

There were other people who had undergone epilepsy surgery, and were pleased to report that they were seizure-free for the first time in years. Some of these lives were changed forever, and for the better. These stories were always welcomed and celebrated.

*Diary entry, Monday, August 8th, 1988*

Today Jesse was fine until about 6:00. I was sitting on the chair by his bed and I just glanced up. There was no warning, no sound. His face seemed contorted. His head was turned to the left and his left eye and mouth were twitching hard. . . .

He went into convulsions, his left arm and leg jerking. He made a sound with each convulsion. His head jerked to the left. He seemed to be awake. His eyes were not rolled. These convulsions went on for what seemed forever—it was only three minutes. His hand was partially closed but it kept on rhythmically jerking open and closed.

After this stopped, his face started to go blotchy red and white and kept turning darker blotches. His left hand was also very blotchy and was paralysed, as was his left leg. This lasted for quite some time afterward. His leg was the first to gain back feeling, and then his arm. He could eventually lift his arm up, but the hand and fingers still drooped. Then the feeling came back in his fingers. . . .

My poor, poor sweet baby! I am so afraid for him. This is truly a horrible disease. I'm so scared and it hurts for me to write about his seizures. But I must keep track. Maybe they will help the doctors to understand better or to help someone else's baby some day.

Dr. Curran said that we could probably go home by the 17th, as long as we can get approval on Cyclosporin from the government. We have not got it yet.

*Diary entry, Friday, August 12, 1988*

Jesse does not look good today. His skin is blotchy. He seems to be very tired, has stomach-aches, and he's shaky. His eyes don't look good. He's very quiet. He's gained so much weight and his face is bloated. I don't like it at all. I don't like these medications, but I don't like the alternative, either. I'm very anxious to get home, but I'm scared as hell to go home. I wish I could be a kid for a week and not have to make decisions. I'm so tired of being scared.

I slept at the hospital that night, as Jesse was having seizures and stomach-aches almost constantly. They gave him Amphogel and Gravol, but it didn't seem to help.

On Saturday I came to the hospital late, having stopped to buy Jesse some pyjamas and an outfit to go home in. None of his clothes fit him any more. He was bloated from the Prednisone, and his appetite had increased as well.

We had a day pass, so when I got to the hospital I thought we might go for a walk. Before we reached the front doors, Jesse had a stomach-ache and changed his mind.

On Sunday we were able to go out. When I opened the doors to the world, it felt as if we had stepped out of a black-and-white picture into living colour. Things were alive, the air was fresh. There were no hospital smells, no moans, no screams. We left the sickness behind for a few hours, and walked down the street hand in hand. I felt euphoric.

Jesse had two seizures, but they were only absences, and he recovered quickly. We walked to the store for a treat and back to the playground at the foot of the hill. When we returned, I called a pizza place I'd seen from the bus.

"Could you deliver a ham and pineapple pizza to the Montreal Neurological Institute?" I asked.

"To *where*?"

"To the Montreal Neurological Institute. The address is—"

"We don't deliver to hospitals."

"Please," I said. "My son has been in here nearly two months and he just wants a pizza. I could meet you at the entrance."

"I don't know." He hesitated. "Just a minute." I heard him speaking to someone in the background, then: "The Neurological Institute?"

"Yes."

He confirmed the address. "You'll be at the front doors?"

"I'll be there," I promised.

"There'll be a five-dollar delivery charge."

"No problem," I said. "How soon can you get here?"

"About forty-five minutes. You *will* be at the front doors?"

"*Yes!*" I said, laughing.

When the pizza arrived, I made a detour to the cafeteria to buy some pop. Ed came for a visit, so we invited him to the party.

After Jesse was asleep for the night, Ed walked me as far as my bus stop. I gave him a hug and thanked him for being our family when our family couldn't be there. He could not have known what a difference he made.

The Saskatchewan Government balked at providing Jesse with Cyclosporin on the prescription drug plan. They had listed it for organ transplant patients for years, but they were unwilling to set a precedent for the costly Cyclosporin as a treatment for Rasmussen's Encephalitis. Late Tuesday morning Dr. Curran arrived with the news that Sandoz, the drug company that manufactures Cyclosporin, had agreed to donate the drug for the one-year trial. He had informed Dr. Lowry in Saskatoon. Now we had only to wait for Saskatchewan Health to approve the drug—which, according to Dr. Lowry, should be no problem. Dr. Curran informed us that we should be able to go home on Thursday. After fifty days and fifty nights in a strange city, I wasted no time in booking the flight for Thursday noon.

We were going home.

# 8 / "What Does a Hot Dog Look Like?"

It was good to be home, though it felt strange at first. Having Chris to help again with Jesse was a blessing for all of us. At the same time, I couldn't help feeling that he was somehow intruding on my territory. Jesse and I had gone to Montreal alone, and we had come back alone. We had shared the most intense experiences a mother and child can have, and we had shared them alone. Everyone else was an outsider.

That night I broke down. It was like a dam bursting, releasing the tensions of the past two months. I cried for Jesse. I cried for his future. I cried for Tara and for Chris. And I cried for myself. I felt as low as I had ever felt, I think, but afterwards it was good to know that I didn't have to hold back any more.

I met with Dr. Lowry soon after we returned. He knew very little about Rasmussen's Encephalitis, and was definitely interested in learning more. I lent him the papers I had been given in Montreal. In return, he gave me a tape of the *Donahue* show that one of his patients had recorded. The guests on the program included several Rasmussen's Encephalitis patients and two doctors who were knowledgeable about the disease.

I watched it the minute the kids were in bed that evening. Then I watched it again, hanging on every word as the patients and their doctors spoke about seizures and hemispherectomies. I looked for clues to the possible outcome and duration of Jesse's illness. The next day I wrote to the network, asking for the addresses of the doctors who had appeared on the program.

Jesse's seizures were as frequent as they had ever been, but he wasn't coming out of them as easily. One day I was alerted to a seizure by the sound of a bowl dropping in the kitchen. Chris carried Jesse to the couch as he began to convulse. When it was over, he tried to get up, but kept falling back. I could see he was paralysed on his left side. He didn't respond to either of us. Finally he stopped trying to get up. His head dropped on the pillow. I looked him right in the eye, and he looked right through me.

"Jesse, can you see Mommy?" I asked. When there was no response, I spoke louder: "JESSE, CAN YOU SEE MOMMY?"

Still there was no response. His blank eyes were staring at nothing that I could see. He was lost. I had to find him and bring him back. It was taking much longer than usual. Again and again I tried to reach him, to no avail.

"Jesse, squeeze my hand."

I closed his fingers around mine, but he couldn't grip.

"Jesse, do you want breakfast?"

If anything could reach him, I thought, that would. Since he had been on steroids, he was constantly hungry. But he only turned to one side and began picking at his clothes. He was alone in a distant room, with a sound-proof wall between us.

I took his chin in my hand and once again looked him in the eye. "Jesse, can you see Mommy?"

After what seemed an eternity, he looked back. But it was the look of a newborn baby. He watched my eyes, then moved his gaze down to my mouth as he became aware that that was where the sounds were coming from—sounds that he didn't seem able to interpret as words. I was afraid, suddenly, that I wouldn't be able to bring him all the way back, that he would stay trapped between the two worlds he seemed to inhabit.

*I'm not going to lose you, honey-bear,* I thought. *Not now. You're almost here. Keep coming.*

At long last, he began to moan in answer to my questions. Slowly, he regained the power of speech. By then the paralysis had gone.

"Do you want breakfast?" I asked.

"Yes," he drawled.

It had been forty-five minutes since the onset of the seizure.

I was concerned about placing Jesse in school. I realized he would have a difficult time keeping up, and I wondered if there were some school in Saskatoon where he might get more individual attention.

Dr. Lowry arranged for us to see a child psychiatrist, Dr. Quinn. He concluded that Jesse should be in a regular classroom, but suggested that there be a resource room available and remedial help when necessary. Jesse's current school, he said, should be able to meet these needs. He asked me to write about the changes I had observed in Jesse:

> Now that we know about Jesse having Rasmussen's Encephalitis, many things have changed. I am still afraid of his seizures, but now I am only afraid that he will not come out of them. I am afraid of the paralysis that follows his *grande mals*. I am afraid to let him go anywhere alone in case he has a seizure and hurts himself, or can't come out of it. I am afraid if he has an absence around other people, they will not recognize it, and may yell at him to answer them when he can't.
>
> Mostly now I am afraid for his future. Some days I still can't accept the physical and mental deterioration that is likely to take place. He will never be completely normal. On the days when I can handle this, I am terrified that I will not handle him properly. My main concern, whether he is mentally or physically handicapped, is that he be happy. I know that I play a major role in his life and am therefore a major factor on which this is decided. I am worried that I may not be able to handle it, that I may not be patient enough, understanding enough, or even compassionate enough for him to be truly happy with the way he is, or the way he becomes. Sometimes I feel I just don't have the strength.
>
> Now that we know there is a reason for his behaviour, it is much easier to be patient with him. But I find that some days this is not enough. Once in a while I still speak to him harshly when he can't remember or do simple things. I think when I act this way I am actually mad at the world for letting this awful thing happen to my Jesse boy.
>
> Mostly I feel sorry for him. For all the things I feel he will be missing in his life. But once in a while I feel sorry for myself, too.
>
> I am worried about Jesse being hurt—not physically, but emotionally, by his peers. I don't want him to feel inadequate or frustrated. So far, he seems to be dealing with his seizures very well. He rarely complains (which, of course, sometimes worries me.)
>
> He doesn't know that he has Rasmussen's Encephalitis. I see no reason to worry him with what may or may not happen in the future. We can't be unrealistic about this disease, yet we must not be pessimistic. There is always room for hope. Meanwhile, a person has to live. Jesse is growing up. I don't want his memories of childhood to be filled with misery.

A woman from the public school board came to see us. She was meant to be a support to parents who had children with problems, but I couldn't figure out what to say to her. The problem was that Jesse was changing. I was losing bits of him that would never return. I didn't understand him. I didn't recognize him any more.

I needed more information. My sister Henriette showed me how to use the computers at the university medical library. Very little has been written about Rasmussen's Encephalitis, but I managed to turn up a few articles. Many nights I went to bed early with these precious papers, reading them over and over until their meaning sank in.

Jesse was gaining so much weight because of the steroid therapy that I had a hard time finding clothes to fit him. His appetite was enormous. He couldn't eat when he was having a bad day, but he made up for it when he was feeling better. I had to laugh when I looked at him in his brown Beavers Club outfit: with his rounded cheeks and belly, his new front teeth looking disproportionately large in his mouth, and the stubble on his head standing upright, he really did look like a beaver.

At the beginning of October, Jesse had another EEG and a CT scan. When we met with Dr. Lowry a few days later, he said that Jesse's EEG still showed some right frontal epileptic discharges. He believed, however, that they were much less frequent than those shown on the pre-operative recordings. There was also some activity in the left hemisphere.

I was afraid to ask him what that meant, but I had to know: "Does that mean that the disease has spread to the other hemisphere?"

"Not necessarily. It may be kindling."

"I don't understand."

"Kindling is residual activity after a seizure. It sometimes crosses over to the other hemisphere."

I left his office praying that was all it was. Kindling.

Jesse's new immunosuppressant medications were being monitored once a week by a nephologist, Dr. Dyck. If the Cyclosporin levels were too high or too low, he would call me with a recommendation to increase or decrease the dosage. The anticonvulsant levels were also being checked, and Dr. Lowry's office followed the same procedure. If no one called, I was to carry on as usual.

We had been warned that, because of these medications, the symptoms of another illness might be absent or masked. I was to have him checked at the first sign of an infection. When Jesse came home from school one day complaining of a sore throat, I took him straight to the hospital, where he was given antibiotics.

We had also been warned that his seizures would increase when he was fighting an infection. So it proved. He spent a restless night, and went into an absence seizure first thing in the morning. After three minutes I put him on the couch, expecting him to fall asleep. Instead, he went into a *grande mal* which lasted another two minutes. Then he finally dozed off. In the next three hours he woke up five times—each time just long enough to have another seizure. After each seizure, he fell back asleep. At noon I woke him up and took him to see Dr. Lowry.

Before Jesse had been diagnosed with Rasmussen's, Dr. Lowry's inability or refusal to do anything to stop the seizures had infuriated me. Time after time I backed the poor man into a corner, but he always came out fighting. When I questioned his methods, or the lack of them, he showed his own frustration, arguing his position as strenuously as I argued mine. Now I still felt the anger, but it wasn't so intense, and it wasn't directed at Dr. Lowry any more. It was directed at the disease. Only Rasmussen's Encephalitis didn't bother arguing its position. It didn't have to. I could rant and rave and question and prod, but the disease silently ignored me and went on wreaking destruction on my child.

Dr. Lowry admitted Jesse to the hospital for observation, and to increase his medication. He slept off and on between seizures and stomach-aches. The myoclonic jerks were almost constant while he slept. I sat by his bedside and timed them. I never got past three seconds before another part of his body twitched. It was the following afternoon before the anticonvulsants made an appreciable difference. After a seizure-free night, Jesse was discharged from hospital. For the next five days he didn't have any seizures, and his stomach-aches were less frequent.

Jesse's intellectual capacity continued to deteriorate. His printing and his drawings became more and more simplified, and his memory was still slipping. One day I asked Jesse and Tara if they wanted chicken or hot dogs for supper. Jesse couldn't remember what a hot dog was. "What does it look like?" he asked. At first I thought he was joking. But it wasn't until I showed him the package that he remembered. He was also forgetting which of his cousins belonged to which aunt and uncle. Incidents like this began to happen often enough that soon they no longer surprised me.

At our next appointment, I told Dr. Lowry that things were not getting better; they were getting worse. Jesse's personality was continuing to change, and he was becoming more difficult to live with. I asked if it was possible if the new drugs were in some way contributing to the behaviour problem. Dr. Lowry wasn't sure, but he promised to check on it. He set up another appointment with the pædiatric psychiatrist.

At Dr. Quinn's request, the school had completed a Connors Rating Scale to measure Jesse's behaviour at school, and I had done one for his behaviour at home. The school also videotaped Jesse for a few hours in class. As an example of "normal" classroom behaviour, it was a laughable failure; it was obvious to everyone that there was nothing normal about moving a student's desk to the side and putting him on camera for the day.

Nevertheless, I didn't have any answers, and I wasn't coping well with Jesse's constant need for attention and his disregard for others. I knew he had lost the ability to plan sequentially, that he could no longer grasp the consequences of his actions, that he acted on the desire of the moment and was unable to learn from past experience. I knew it didn't matter how many times he was reprimanded or sent to his room. I knew his behaviour was getting worse as the disease advanced through his brain, and that none of these things was his fault. I knew it in my heart and in my mind, yet after a day, a week, a month of this kind of behaviour, it was impossible to rationalize. His impulsiveness was driving me crazy.

The results of the Connors Rating Scale and the videotape confirmed Dr. Quinn's diagnosis that Jesse was suffering from an Attention Deficit/ Hyperactivity disorder (ADHD): "It's likely that a lot of this is due to the surgery. When children undergo brain surgery, it often takes a full year for them to completely recover. Many things can go on within that year until they become themselves again."

"But this behaviour didn't start after the surgery." I argued. "It began shortly after the onset of his seizures. Maybe some of it's due to the surgery, but his impulsiveness and distractibility are a continuation of what was happening when the seizures began. It's just becoming more consistent and more visible."

"What was he like before the seizures?" he asked.

I took a breath, and smiled as I recalled my old Jesse. "He was totally different. He was bright, easy going, likable. We've been watching his personality change almost since the seizures first appeared. I'm sure it's the disease that's causing the behaviour difficulties." I wondered, too, if the medications were at least partly responsible. He'd been on anticonvulsants since the seizures began, and now he was taking steroids and immuno-suppressants as well. I certainly didn't believe the ADHD was due to the surgery. In fact, I had trouble believing the whole diagnosis. I didn't realize that ADHD, like epilepsy, is a symptom, not a disease.

Dr. Quinn was patient. "Whatever the cause," he said, "I recommend that you read these." He handed me a book and some literature. "It will help you to understand ADHD better. I'd also like you to consider putting Jesse on Ritalin. I've found it to be beneficial to many of my patients."

I shook my head decisively. "I won't put him on any more drugs, especially not one that's designed to alter his thinking and behaviour even more."

"Take the literature anyway," he said. "After you've read it, if you have any questions, we can discuss them. Then, if you still feel the same way, I'll respect your decision."

I agreed to read the literature, but I was determined not to change my mind. My determination began to weaken, however, when I learned that Ritalin wouldn't change Jesse's thinking. It would just help to keep his thoughts organized and focused, and enable him to regain some self-control.

Dr. Lowry thought it was worth a try: "The best thing about Ritalin is that it's quickly metabolized. This makes it a very good trial drug because, if it works, the effects will be visible within days. On the other hand, if there's no change, Jesse can be taken off it without any complications."

I didn't know what to do. I had tried to be patient with Jesse. But it had been two long years, and things were getting worse. Dr. Andermann's words—"He's still in the very early stages of the illness"—kept running through my mind. How many more stages of hell were there?

*Diary entry, January 16th, 1989*
> Jesse's not growing up. Not maturing, not anything. Most of the time,
> I am either so mad or depressed I don't care. I feel like I am slipping
> away. I must get a grip on this—it's scary.

On February 8th, I wrote to Dr. Andermann in Montreal, telling him about Jesse's deteriorating social and intellectual capacities, and asking him to send me any more information, in any form, that he had on Rasmussen's Encephalitis. I also asked him for the names of other parents whose children suffered from Rasmussen's, and told him he could give them my name in return. I asked for his opinions on Ritalin, hemispherectomy, and the prolonged use of anticonvulsants, among other things. "We need some answers," I told him. "We are having a very difficult time coping." I closed by thanking him in advance for answering my letter.

*Letter to Dr. Hwang, Toronto Sick Children's Hospital, February 8th, 1989*
> I have read your report about the six children with Rasmussen's and
> their ongoing medical struggle. One of the cases in this report was
> somewhat similar to my son Jesse's, who also has a slowly progres-
> sive deterioration. I really would like to contact the parents of these
> children and others whose children have Rasmussen's. Jesse's is the
> first diagnosed case in Saskatchewan. We are desperate for any infor-
> mation or comments you may have.

I don't really see a point to keeping these children on large doses of anticonvulsants. As suggested by your paper, much of the mental dullness could be attributed to the large doses of anticonvulsants. Do they do any good at all?

Going over my diary, I discovered what might be a clue to Jesse's behaviour. Things seemed to have started getting out of hand when he began taking Tegretol. I called Dr. Lowry to see what he thought. He hadn't heard of Tegretol interfering with behaviour, and wasn't much taken with my idea. But I was insistent. If Jesse could be maintained on one anticonvulsant instead of the two that he was on, one drug—and, presumably, its side effects—could be eliminated. Dr. Lowry reluctantly agreed, and gave me a protocol for decreasing the dose.

By the end of the month, the seizures flared up again. Doris Newmeyer called from Dr. Lowry's office to say that, because I was reducing the Tegretol, the level of Depakene in Jesse's blood had dropped. Dr. Lowry wanted me to increase the dosage of Depakene. I complied, and Jesse had two seizure-free weeks. Then on March 10th, he had eight seizures. The next day he had twelve.

Dr. Lowry was away, so I spoke to Dr. Sundaram. He told me flatly to increase the Tegretol. I was disappointed. I also felt guilty. Was I responsible for this bout of seizures? There hadn't been enough time to test my theory about the effect of Tegretol on Jesse's behaviour. That would have to be abandoned for now.

Late the next morning, after eleven seizures, I spoke to Dr. Lowry. He pointed out, unnecessarily, that reducing Jesse's Tegretol was evidently not the answer to his behavioural problems. I was to increase it again, gradually, until he was on a maintenance dose of 800 milligrams a day. At my request, Dr. Lowry wrote to Dr. Andermann for a reassessment of the immunosuppressant therapy, and advice as to its continuation.

By the next day, Jesse insisted he felt well enough to go to school. His teacher later called to inform me that he'd had two small absences, but he was fine and wanted to stay at school.

The following day I received a reply from Dr. Hwang in Toronto. He said that without having had a chance to see Jesse, he could not answer my questions about his prognosis. Perhaps I should consult Jesse's pædiatric neurologist in Saskatoon. (*Right,* I thought, *why didn't I think of that?*) Due to the confidentiality of medical information, it would not be possible for him to release the names of any of the cases he had cited in his article. "I thank you for your interest," he concluded, "and will be pleased to see Jesse, if you think I can be of any help. Please ask his pædiatrician or neurologist to write me regarding his medical condition at present."

I was furious. I needed information. I needed *answers*. I was hanging from a cliff by the tips of my fingers, pleading for help, and all the good doctor could do was ask me to whistle him a tune while I hung on.

I hadn't received any answer from the *Donahue* show, either, and had written again about six weeks later. Now another six weeks had passed. There were things the doctors had said on that program that really bothered me. Again, I needed *answers*. So I played the tape again and again until I was satisfied that I had as much information about those two doctors as it was going to give me. Then, using investigative skills I didn't know I had, I came up with a phone number for each of them.

The first doctor made it clear that he wasn't interested in speaking to me. He told me that Dr. Andermann was extremely knowledgeable on the subject, and I should contact him if I needed more information about my son's case. I anticipated a similar response from the second doctor, John Freeman, who worked out of Johns Hopkins Hospital in Baltimore. I called the hospital and managed to get his address. I wrote to him, giving a brief description of Jesse's history and quoting the statements from the *Donahue* show that needed clarification. I felt this letter was my last chance at finding the answers I desperately needed.

A few days later, we took Jesse to a church in Saskatoon where a renowned guest speaker was holding a healing service. I wanted a miracle. I was scared and weary. I was tired of hurting. I wanted a miracle for Jesse, a miracle for me. And I wanted it *now*.

Later that night, I crept into Jesse's room, knelt at his bedside, and laid my hand on his shoulder. The twitching continued. I cried silently onto his blanket. Was my faith not strong enough, or was it not the right time?

The next day, Jesse's teacher called to tell me he had had a seizure. A few days later I noticed him watching television with one eye closed again. I called his teacher, who told me he had been doing the same thing in school for the past few days.

"This is a definite sign of toxicity," I said. "He's overdosing on the medication. If this or anything else unusual happens again, let me know."

I called Dr. Lowry. He agreed that Jesse was likely toxic because of the increases of Tegretol. I was to bring him in for a blood level and reduce the Tegretol by 100 milligrams. The decrease meant, of course, that within twenty-four hours he would be having more seizures.

I was drained. I wanted someone to take over. If only I could be on a tag team, I thought, be a consultant for a while instead of the CEO. I wanted Chris to say, "I'll take over, I'll handle it for you." But he didn't. If he'd tried, he would have done things his way, not mine, and I suspect it wouldn't have been good enough for me.

*Letter received from Dr. John Freeman, March 28th, 1989*
Dear Mrs. Armstrong:

Thank you for your letter of March 15th about your son Jesse. It is a very perceptive letter and I will try to answer your questions.

1) Montreal is one of the premier epilepsy surgery centers in the world. Their experience goes back long before ours and indeed they probably have done more hemispherectomies than we have. So, I think you are in excellent hands.

2) There is no established treatment for Rasmussen's. There are different biases and prejudices but there is no right way to treat it. I personally do not believe that the immunosuppression program that they are using will work, but that is my bias. I do not know the results of their studies.

3) Regarding hemispherectomy, there is indeed debate about how much brain should be taken out, and when a hemispherectomy should be done. We, at Hopkins, are in this case, more radical in doing a hemispherectomy earlier than the group at Montreal. But, Montreal also does them earlier than many other places.

4) I don't have enough information to know if this is Rasmussen's, but, if indeed it is, I think you should consider a hemispherectomy. When that should be done is a matter of opinion and one would have to have a clear idea of how much his intellectual function is declining, and at what rate, or whether it has just stabilized at a lower rate. We do not require a total hemiplegia prior to surgery, but certainly a hemiparesis would be created if surgery was done, and it's hard for people to accept unless there is already some evidence of hemipareses.

In regard to your questions, yes, if this is Rasmussen's, the disease is indeed confined to one hemisphere.

Regarding the younger the patient the easier it is to transfer function, I think this is true. This is particularly true when speech is involved which is not the case with Jesse, but whether younger means 8 or 10, I don't think anybody knows if there is any difference.

We do believe that most children with Rasmussen's lose intellectual function and we have seen it come back with surgery. This is one reason why we like to do it earlier.

Unfortunately, there are no clear answers to when surgery should be done. As far as some showing physical deterioration and some showing more emotional and mental, this is determined by the lobe of the brain that the seizures start in, and by the rapidity of the progression.

I hope this answers your questions. If you would like to talk with our coordinator, Ms. Diana Pillas, I'm sure she can answer some of your questions even better and perhaps put you in touch with somebody from our parent's group.

Sincerely,
John M. Freeman, MD
Professor of Neurology & Pediatrics
The Johns Hopkins Hospital

In March that year we bought a three-bedroom bungalow three blocks from the trailer court and only four blocks from school. It was a blessing to be in a house of our own again. It needed a lot of renovations, but for us, at least one dream had come true.

# 9 / The Best Course of Action?

It was a relief to have Dr. Freeman confirm that Rasmussen's Encephalitis is confined to one hemisphere. As for his doubts about the immuno-suppression program, they didn't surprise me; we had already concluded that that wasn't the answer. For the first time I began, tentatively, to think about hemispherectomy.

Dr. Freeman had answered some of my questions. There were others that remained unanswered, somewhere between here and Dr. Andermann's office in Montreal. I called Faye, his secretary, to find out if he had received my letter. She said she would check.

I called Diana Pillas, as Dr. Freeman had suggested, for I was anxious to get in touch with other parents of children with Rasmussen's. Diana spoke with an air of confidence, and her willingness to help was both obvious and welcome. She gave me the address of a family in Connecticut—Kathy and Brian Usher, and their daughter, Beth—who were willing to discuss their experience.

I wrote to the Ushers immediately, giving them a brief description of the progress of Jesse's illness. I asked about the nature of Beth's deterioration and how they had survived each day. I also asked about the factors on which they had based their decision to have a hemispherectomy performed, and of course I asked about the results of the surgery.

By the end of April, Jesse was still having one or two seizures a day, sometimes more, and they knocked the starch out of him. Sometimes he slept away the better part of a day. On the last Sunday in April, he was only conscious for a few minutes after each seizure. He would wake up and start to eat, only to be interrupted by another seizure. By 3:00 PM he'd had seven seizures and managed to eat half a piece of toast.

Finally I gave him an Ativan—always my last resort—which left him dopey and unsteady, but at least it kept the seizures away for a couple of hours. I was able to coax him to eat part of a hamburger, but after he had another seizure I put him to bed. "It's okay, Honey-bear," I whispered, "you'll have a better day tomorrow."

The next day I received a reply from Kathy Usher. "Received your letter today," she wrote, "and I'm sorry for all that you have gone through. Jesse's illness sounds so much like the beginning of Beth's."

The *beginning*? There it was again. *Lord, how will Jesse survive? How will our family stay together?*

Beth had had her first seizure in kindergarten, and they continued for a year and a half. By that time her right side was weak, especially her arm, and she had become left-handed; she had run the gamut of medications; she had deteriorated mentally and socially, and was beginning to lose her right visual field.

They took Beth to Johns Hopkins to consult with Dr. Freeman. He recommended a left hemispherectomy. He was well informed on Rasmussen's Encephalitis, and the neurosurgeon, Dr. Carson, was experienced in performing the surgery. Dr. Freeman considered this was the best course of action. It was, in fact, the only course that would halt the destruction. In his experience, the removal of only that portion of the brain where the seizures originated arrested neither the seizures nor the disease. Even so, Kathy and Brian decided that they could never do such a thing to their child. They returned home, where the seizures became more frequent and the deterioration accelerated. Finally, in February 1987, two years after her first seizure, Beth Usher was admitted to Johns Hopkins Hospital, where a left hemispherectomy was performed by Dr. Carson.

With the left side of her brain gone, Beth no longer had an occipital lobe to decipher what her eyes were seeing in the right visual field. She had therefore suffered a total loss of her right visual field. Because the left side of the brain controls the right side of the body, she also suffered a right hemiparesis. With time and therapy, she was able to walk again, but her right arm remained of little use, and her hand would always be paralysed. These deficits were a direct result of the surgery, not a complication of it. Beth had already begun to lose her right visual field as well as the strength on that side of her body prior to surgery. What the surgery did was complete the destruction—in return for the hope of stopping the seizures and saving the good hemisphere from interference of function. There were some complications from surgery, but Beth recovered well, and was taken off all anticonvulsants. For two years she had remained seizure free. "This whole ordeal has been a nightmare," Kathy concluded:

> We feel so fortunate that all has worked out so well for us. I will always wonder how this happened. I guess what did keep us going was that we had to get Beth well, no matter what it took. Someone told me that it was our duty as parents to do what was medically possible at this time. So many times, I thought I would lose my mind, but I would try to learn more and more about the disease and make sure that Beth was always happy.
>
> I knew that her prior behaviour and illness were not her fault, but it was hard trying to be a normal family. Our son Brian, aged twelve, was older and able to understand that we had a major problem. He tried to help, but I'm sure he suffered in many ways. Looking back, it seems like surgery was a hundred years ago.

I felt a profound closeness to Beth's family. Their letter gave me comfort and hope. It also raised more questions, and hastened my need for answers. Jesse had been under attack for over two and a half years now, and there was still no sign of hemiparesis or a loss of visual field. Did that mean that much of that hemisphere was still intact after hundreds of seizures, or was the temporal lobe that contained the motor strip all that was left? I wondered, too, how much the damaged hemisphere was interfering with the healthy one.

"Jesse." It was Chris. He was giving Jesse a bath. Jesse was probably having a seizure. If it was an emergency, Chris would have called me. Nevertheless, I went to them. I had to be there, even if Chris was handling it. Jesse was in an absence. Chris had his arms around him in case he went into convulsions. Not this time, thank God. He was groggy when he came out of it, but he was able to continue his bath.

The next day my sister Yvonne came to visit. We walked to school to meet the kids. On our way back, Jesse stopped in the middle of the road and stared. As usual, I asked him if he was okay. He turned his head to the left. The left side of his mouth began to twitch, and his eyes were jerking to the left. It became more rapid. I held him in case he went into convulsions, and I spoke to him calmly and steadily: "It's okay, Honey. It's okay, Jesse." I felt sympathy and regret, but my fear of seizures was gone.

In the last month Jesse had lost weight because of his stomach-aches, but he was still overweight from the steroids. I wasn't sure I'd be able to carry him home. I stopped wondering about that when his left leg went up.

Convulsions were only seconds away. I scooped him up and ran. We made it to the front lawn of our house before I had to put him down. I told Yvonne to get Chris. Chris carried him into the house and put him on his bed, where Jesse convulsed for another two minutes. I wasn't afraid any more, but it still bruised my heart to see him like this.

I pulled off his shoes and positioned his paralysed arm and leg so they wouldn't be uncomfortable when the feeling came back. "You okay, Jesse?" He nodded slightly, eyes closed. I pulled the covers over him, and closed the door as I left.

*Safe for this time,* I thought. *But what about next time? Will I be there, or will he smash his head on the pavement?*

Dr. Lowry said to increase the Tegretol to 800 milligrams a day. That was the level at which he began showing symptoms of toxicity.

Since Dr. Andermann never returned my calls, I asked Chris to call him. It had been three and a half months since I wrote, pleading for answers. Chris managed to get through.

"Did he get my letter?" I asked, afterward.

"Yes, but he told me he had no intention of answering it. He—"

"What!" I interrupted.

"He said he would have to see Jesse before he could answer your questions. He thinks we should have a re-evaluation done. He said to have Dr. Lowry call him and he'll put Jesse on the waiting list in Montreal."

My questions had been about Rasmussen's in general and hemispherectomy in particular. He didn't have to see Jesse in order to pass on information about the disease. I had told him we were desperate. I had described Jesse's condition. And I'd waited three months for a letter *he had no intention of answering.* I was shocked and furious. I called Dr. Lowry immediately and, as calmly as I could, asked him to write or call Dr. Andermann to request a re-evaluation.

By the end of May Jesse was seeing double again. He was walking into walls and having four or five seizures a day, sleeping between times. In June he got an ear infection and was put on antibiotics. More drugs. His blood levels indicated the Tegretol was in the high range. I walked into Dr. Lowry's office, holding Jesse by the hand so he wouldn't fall against the walls.

Dr. Lowry examined him. "His visual fields are still intact," he commented, "and there is no evidence of left-sided weakness. I see he's a bit groggy."

"Groggy and very unsteady," I said. "He walks into walls. His appetite has diminished. He has frequent stomach-aches. He turns down treats now, and he's losing weight. I'm worried. Something has to be done."

Dr. Lowry thought a moment. "I'd like to try Tegretol CR," he said. "It's released consistently into the blood steam, so there aren't the peaks and valleys you get from most medications. We might be able to maintain the same blood levels with a smaller dosage, and hopefully gain seizure control without the toxicity. We could maintain him on this medication on 600 milligrams a day."

"It's worth a try." The sky was still falling on Jesse, but at least Dr. Lowry was trying to find something to support him. "What about the last EEG?"

"There seems to be more activity. The involvement from the other side seems to be increasing, too."

I felt the familiar stab of fear. "What does that mean?"

"As I've said before, it may just be kindling from the right hemisphere."

"But what if it's not? Even if the disease doesn't spread to the left hemisphere, could it be developing a focal point there? What the hell are we going to do if the disease destroys his right hemisphere and in the process creates a focal point for seizures in the left?"

"I can't say," said Dr. Lowry. "The literature suggests that it doesn't involve the contra-lateral hemisphere, so I assume the activity is kindling."

"But we have to know!" I protested.

"I agree," he responded. "But I don't have enough experience with this syndrome. You'll have to ask Dr. Andermann in Montreal."

"Have you heard from him yet?"

"No, but I'm going to a conference in Ottawa this week and I expect to see him there. I'll ask him when he'll be able to get Jesse in for a re-evaluation."

*Soon!* I pleaded. *Let it be soon!*

When I tried to fill the prescription for Tegretol CR—the CR stands for "controlled release"—the pharmacist informed me that it was not on the prescription plan. I was to call my doctor and he could fill out the appropriate forms. Doris in Dr. Lowry's office said she would take care of it immediately, but it would take a week or two to go through.

Jesse, meanwhile, continued to see double. He felt sick to his stomach, and couldn't eat. Even so, he vomited during the night. I reduced his Tegretol by 100 milligrams the following day. We would simply have to deal with the increase in seizures.

I took him grocery shopping with me. He didn't want to go. He said it took too much energy to walk. I thought it would be good for him to see his favourite foods. His appetite, I naïvely reasoned, might return.

"That'll be $68.45," the clerk said.

Jesse clutched his stomach. I watched him out of the corner of my eye to see if it would develop into a seizure. The clerk waited. Jesse's eyes glazed over. I put down my pen and closed my cheque book. He didn't respond when I spoke to him. His left arm bent at the elbow and the hand began to cup. This was a new type of seizure.

I turned to the clerk who was looking impatiently to the line of customers behind me.

"He's having a seizure," I said. "We'll have to wait a minute."

I prayed that a minute was all it would take, that he wouldn't go into convulsions, that he would be spared the emotional pain of having everyone gawk at him. I was long past the point of being embarrassed about creating a scene in public, but I hated people looking at him as if he were an injured animal. And I was angry at the people in line who were manœuvring to get a better look at the boy who was having a seizure.

Everyone waited.

No one said a word.

Within a minute the seizure had passed. He began to sway, barely able to keep his eyes open. I scooped up his slackened body and set him in the shopping cart. "You okay, honey-bear?" I asked.

"Un-hunh," he whispered before he fell asleep.

I picked up my pen and began writing the cheque as if nothing had happened.

On June 26th I was able to fill the prescription for Tegretol CR. It was a straight exchange of medication without having to decrease one and slowly increase the other.

Dr. Lowry returned from Ottawa. He had seen Dr. Andermann, and Dr. Andermann had promised to put Jesse on his emergency list.

Jesse's ear infection seemed to be hanging on. Our GP put him on a different antibiotic.

A few days later a call came from Montreal. We were to be at the hospital for Monday, July 24th. I filled out another application to the Kinsmen Foundation. Two days later we were accepted. I made airline reservations.

My sister Jeanne insisted that she babysit the kids so that Chris and I could have some time together before I went to Montreal. The week-end of July 8th, we went on a holiday. But we were hardly alone. There were twelve of us, family and friends, at Otter Rapids. We slept in tents, and cooked over an open fire. We fished as the sun was going down, then sat by the fire singing songs and telling jokes. For a day and a half I barely thought of my responsibilities. I pretended I was like the rest of them, a normal person with a normal life.

The next day brought me back to reality. Shooting the rapids in inner tubes proved more challenging than we were prepared for—or maybe we just weren't prepared. We had three near-mishaps. No one was hurt, but the six-hour drive home gave me time to think. It was then that it hit me.

I had never thought of dying, but now it loomed large. I couldn't die. It was as simple as that. I had to look after Jesse. I could not tempt fate again. I couldn't take chances, however slight—not until I got Jesse through this. I would have traded my life for his health in a moment, but I wasn't offered that bargain. It was living for him that was hard. Seizures rob their victims of all control, so someone has to take control for them. Someone has to be there.

Shortly after our trip to Otter Rapids, I began to have another nightmare. My life in the dream was the same as it was in reality. Jesse had seizures and I was responsible for him. Then, late one night, I found Chris in a seizure. The feeling of desolation was absolute. I would die rather than take on one more responsibility. But I couldn't die. I woke up feeling weak and defeated. The pillow was wet with tears, and I was still crying. I realized it was only a dream, but it kept coming back, and each time it was as real as the first.

On July 23rd, Chris drove Jesse and Tara and me to the Saskatoon airport. Tara was to stay in Toronto with her grandparents while Jesse and I flew on to Montreal.

We arrived at four o'clock. I had arranged to stay at the same boarding house I had stayed at last year. Jesse was to stay with me the first night, and would be admitted to the Neurological Institute the following day.

The heat was almost unbearable. Jesse slept in his shorts on a mattress on the floor while I lay awake on the bed in my panties and t-shirt, listening to the traffic sounds and the sirens, and to Jesse's occasional moans. I crept down onto the mattress with him. I could feel his body twitching. What would it take, I wondered, to subdue this inner battle?

# 10 / Montreal *Encore*

*D*iary entry, July 24th, 1989

I called the hospital today. They said a doctor wanted to speak to me. He said the resident under Dr. Andermann was sick and he would not admit us until the resident was back at work, which might be Tuesday or Wednesday. I was really PO'd, and I thought about it all day. Finally I called Dr. Andermann's office. Faye said she would speak to Dr. Andermann about it. She did. He said he would personally admit us on Tuesday or Wednesday.

Thank you so much! So here we sit, 33° outside and about 50° in here. More humidity than Montreal has ever seen. Having a great time! Wish you were here! The only consolation is that Jesse hasn't had any seizures today. Many jerks, but no seizures.

Jesse was admitted at 3:00 PM the following day. Walking up the familiar steps and into the foyer, my feelings were mixed. Part of me felt a sense of foreboding. Another part looked forward to the possibility of answers to our problems.

We were taken to our old room. The construction crew outside the window was gone, but everything else was the same. Dr. Andermann's new resident came in to take our history. She looked harried.

The following day, Wednesday, Jesse had three seizures. One of them was a type he had recently acquired. He would stare for a few seconds, and then laugh. He might be tired after one of these, but sometimes he wasn't. Where in the brain is the funny bone? I wondered.

Another type of seizure, brief but frequent, also began around this time. He would stop dead in his tracks, tilt to the left for a couple of seconds, and then shake his head—to "shake it out," as he called it.

I took him down to EEG at 2:00 o'clock. We were anxious to see Francine again. Peter, who had been there last year, told us that she had moved to another hospital. He would call her, though, because he knew she would be anxious to see us.

On Thursday I finally saw Dr. Andermann. He walked into the room, his entourage two paces behind him. "Hello, Mrs. Armstrong. How are you?"

"Hello, Dr. Andermann. We're fine, thanks. Jesse's—"

"He looks well," he interrupted. "I know you have many questions, and that is rightly so. But first we have to do more testing to see how much he has deteriorated. Then we will discuss the results. I will speak with you more later."

I had come too far and waited too long to let him get away that easily. "The EEG shows seizure activity in the left hemisphere," I said. "What does that mean?"

"Don't worry about it for now. We will speak to Dr. Antel, the nephologist, and Dr. Taylor, the psychologist. First, I would like to see his EEG for myself."

Up went the stop sign. Time was up.

We met again the following day. He had eliminated Cyclosporin from Jesse's treatment, but kept him on Imuran and Prednisone.

"I've kept track of Jesse's seizures," I told him. "The *grande mals* have been fewer, but the absences have increased. He's also been having a number of smaller seizures and arm jerks that he didn't have last year. As far as I can see, this program has been a failure. I don't see any point in continuing with it."

"I'm not sure this is totally true," Dr. Andermann countered. "I think we would have seen much more deterioration had he not been on the program. I would agree, however, that it doesn't seem to have been as successful as I had hoped."

"You talked about surgery once the neurologic status has stabilized," I said. "When would that happen?"

"It varies with each patient. It usually happens when a maximal hemiparesis and total visual field loss has occurred. This may be anywhere from one to twenty years."

*Twenty years! God help us.*

"Does the part of the brain that has atrophied or died still seize until it is removed?"

"The seizures will continue even after stabilization," he replied. "It is only when the hemisphere is removed that the patient has a good chance of becoming seizure free."

"Then why not just remove the portion of the brain that seems to be affected? The EEG shows that Jesse's seizures seem to be coming from the frontal lobe. It obviously hasn't destroyed his motor strip or his occipital lobe. Won't removing the frontal lobe stop both the seizures and the spread of the disease?"

"That has been tried, but it produced only a moderate reduction in seizures in some patients. In others it made little or no difference. This type of surgery carried out early in the course of the disease does not aggravate the inflammatory process, but it is clearly ineffective in protecting the patient from further deterioration."

I asked if it was true, as I had heard the doctors on *Donahue* say, that "very rarely do you find a case where only the right or left hemisphere is damaged."

"This is true of many brain diseases," he replied. "But not with Rasmussen's. One of the classic features of Rasmussen's Encephalitis is its lateralization to one hemisphere."

Then I asked a question that had puzzled me for some time: "Why didn't you suspect Rasmussen's when we first came here last year?"

"I believe it was because he was in the earliest stages of the disease. I think we will have a better idea next week, after the test results come back. We can talk more then."

I called Ed's number, but he had moved. Jesse and I were both disappointed, but Francine came the next evening. She said she was working on Saturday, but insisted on taking us out Sunday and spending the day with us. I didn't resist.

I went up to the third-floor lounge. All the regulars were gone, except Norman. I smiled at him and said hello. He smiled back, but he obviously didn't remember me. What must it be like, I wondered, to live only in the present? Perhaps his life was not as bleak and melancholy as I had once imagined. For a moment I almost envied him.

I saw another familiar face. "How are you?"

"Not too bad." Recognition lit up his eyes. "You were here last year with your little boy. Are you having more problems?"

"We're here for a re-evaluation," I said. "You haven't been here all this time, have you?" *What a stupid question,* I thought, as soon as I had uttered it. What if he had been? I hoped he was only in for a check-up.

"No, no. I was having a problem with my shunt. They changed it."

More shop talk. Shunts. Brain surgery. Seizures. Tumours. Then, from a corner of the room, I heard, "You know, there's a man on Three West that has AIDS."

"No!" came the reply.

"Yes. They keep his door shut most of the time. The nurses go in with masks and gloves. They say he's near the end."

"I don't know why they have to bring those people here."

"His wife comes to visit, but she looks horrid. They say she has the virus, too. He gave it to her."

"They shouldn't be allowed. They should have their own place."

How do we justify thinking one illness inferior to another? I wondered. There's no book listing the highest to lowest in terms of dignity and self-worth. Is it because we are forced to face our own mortality when we are faced with another's illness?

For centuries epileptics faced rejection and disdain. As late as the nineteenth century epilepsy was regarded in some quarters as demonic possession. Far into the twentieth century its victims were being held in psychiatric facilities. Some epileptics came to believe that they actually were evil. Many more believed their illness was something to be ashamed of, and tried to hide it. Even medical students have been taught to shun the term. A 1985 edition of a leading text advised, "The word epilepsy still has unpleasant connotations, and is probably best avoided in dealing with patients until such time as the general public becomes more enlightened." In the meantime, the epileptic walks a lonely road, knowing there's a sniper lying in wait. The sniper gives no warning—other than the certainty that somewhere, some time, he is going to open fire.

We had a day pass on the weekend, so we spent Saturday afternoon away from the hospital. It was only a few blocks from the Institute to Sherbrooke Street and Boulevard de Maisonneuve, and a block further to *rue* Ste-Catherine in downtown Montreal. I looked forward to the break. Jesse wasn't as excited as I thought he would be. He really wasn't interested in walking that far, but I insisted, and ended up bribing him with the promise of seeing a movie.

It was hot and humid, but we arrived on busy St. Catherine Street with only one rest stop along the way. I pointed out the historic buildings to Jesse, their stone walls covered in lush vines. But he wasn't interested. "How much longer, Mom?" was all he wanted to know. We soon found a theatre with "Now Playing: Babar" on the marquee. It's hard to say which of us enjoyed the movie more. Jesse loved the artwork and the story, and it was a joy for me to see him laughing and munching junk food just like any other kid.

On Sunday morning, Francine took us to her house. She had a swimming pool in the yard, and she and Jesse played in it for a couple of hours. I basked in the sun and took delight in Jesse's laughter. He didn't have a single seizure.

Later Francine took us sight-seeing, but Jesse quickly became bored. He wasn't interested in where the Expos played, or in any of the other things that most boys his age would marvel at. He had lost interest in anything that fell outside his immediate range of attention. So Francine took us to a park where we played with Jesse on the swings and in the sand. Then we went for supper to a little Chinese restaurant. The smorgasbord looked delicious. It had the tiniest drumsticks I had ever seen. I placed some on my plate and some on Jesse's. When we were sitting down, I picked one up and began to eat.

"These are delicious, Francine," I said. "I've never seen such small chicken."

Jesse was enjoying his, too, gobbling each one in a single bite.

"It's not chicken," Francine said. "It's *la grenouille*. . . . How do you say that in English?" She thought a minute, annoyed with herself for not knowing the English word. "You know, they are green and small."

I tried to think of a small chicken with green feathers. "A cornish hen?" I asked, munching the delicate meat.

"No." She shook her head. "Oh, I just forget the word. . . . You know, they go hop, hop, hop."

*Hop, hop, hop,* I thought, a fresh "drumstick" halfway to my mouth. "Not a frog?"

"Yes, yes! That's it, frog's legs."

I dropped the little leg from my fingers.

"What, you don't like it?" asked Francine as she saw the stricken look on my face.

"I can't eat a frog," I said simply, pushing them off to the side of my plate.

"Can I have them?" asked Jesse.

"Sure," I replied.

We changed the topic and continued our meal. Jesse went for more frog's legs. I stuck to chow mein, rice, and Chinese vegetables. We returned to the hospital only minutes before our day pass expired.

The week went by slowly. The days were hot and very, very long. Jesse had an MRI on Wednesday, and slept for most of the day from the sedative. I spoke to a neuro-psychologist about Jesse's behavioural problems and the regression, but we couldn't accomplish much in one session.

At my next meeting with Dr. Andermann, he suggested a program of treatment they were trying in France. It involved high doses of Prednisone. I didn't like that idea at all.

"The initial results look promising," he said.

"At our last meeting," I reminded him, " you said it might be twenty years before Jesse is ready for hemispherectomy. He can't stay on steroids for twenty years. There must be another option."

"Jesse is still far too high functioning to consider hemispherectomy," he responded. "In the meantime, this program holds the most promise."

"How do we know when it's time?"

The stop sign went up. "I will arrange for you to see our neurosurgeon, Dr. Villemure. He has done all our modified hemispherectomies since Dr. Rasmussen retired." He handed me an article entitled "High Dose Steroid Treatment of Epilepsia Partialis Continua Due to Chronic Focal Encephalitis," and again urged me to consider the program.

Dr. Villemure was pleasant, and I felt at ease with him. I told him what Dr. Freeman had said about Montreal doing hemispherectomies later than Johns Hopkins, but "earlier than many other places." I wanted to know what that meant; specifically, what it meant for Jesse. But Dr. Villemure echoed Dr. Andermann. It was much too early to consider hemispherectomy: "Jesse hasn't yet begun to lose the left visual field. More importantly, he's had no left-sided weakness as yet."

"When do we know it's time?"

"We don't require a total hemiparesis prior to surgery, as some other hospitals do, but there should at least be a weakness progressing into a hemiparesis. A hemiparesis would definitely occur after surgery, and other functions would be lost as well. No one can say how much function is still operative in the right hemisphere. We know his motor strip is unaffected at this point because he can still move his left limbs, but other, more subtle, functions are also still operating, functions we can't detect with a scan. Once a hemispherectomy is performed, all those functions are lost. Forever."

I had a final conference with Dr. Andermann on Friday. He again urged me to try the high-dose steroids for a year. The long-term side effects would be minimal, he said; there was a slight chance of contracting leukemia. In the short term, there would be an increase in appetite and perhaps a slight weight gain. He would send the protocol to Dr. Lowry.

I asked more specific questions about the program, but he had no concrete evidence of its effectiveness. All he could say was that it looked promising. I said I would discuss it with Chris and we would think about it.

At 8:00 PM, a doctor walked into our room as I was getting Jesse ready for bed. He introduced himself as Dr. Matthews, and asked if he could speak to me outside the room. Curious and apprehensive, I followed him to a small waiting room down the hall.

"I have been studying the chemistry of the cells in Rasmussen's Encephalitis for some time," he began. "Through repeated MRIs we are trying to identify the chemistry of the encephalitic cells, determine how and why they are changing, and what happens to them as they change. We hope in this way to find the etiology of the syndrome.

"Your son," he continued, "is in the beginning stages of the disease. Other children I have studied have all been in the latter stages. I believe Jesse may be a benefit to further our studies. Comparing his brain cells to those of a child in the latter stages may give us clues as to how and why the cells are changing, and possibly bring us closer to a cure."

"We're going home tomorrow," I said. There was no changing my mind on that. In any case, I didn't want to put Jesse through more tests.

"I realize that, and it's already getting late. I apologize for the hastiness of my request, but I only learned today that you were leaving tomorrow. I have arranged to use the MRI later this evening. I would certainly appreciate your permission to do the test, but let me say that it is purely for research. It isn't required for his treatment."

"I'm certainly concerned about finding a cure for this disease," I said, "if not for Jesse, then for the children who come after him. But he's been through so much already. Tell me exactly what you want to do."

"The test will take just over an hour, and he needs to be asleep. That means a sedative, unfortunately, and a needle."

Jesse didn't mind needles, but in my opinion he had enough of them that were necessary without volunteering for more. "Is there any danger?" I asked, looking for a way out.

"Not any more than there would be with a regular MRI. I understand your concern, and your hesitation. I'm sure your son has been put through plenty of necessary tests, so your reluctance to agree to this one is understandable."

I wished he would stop being so understanding and nice. It would have been easy to say no to someone who was pushy.

"I'll ask Jesse," I said, at length. "It will have to be up to him. If he agrees, then I'll give you my permission."

"Thank you." He handed me a card. "You can call me at this number when you've reached a decision."

I told Jesse about Dr. Matthews' request. He asked if he had to have that needle again, the one in the hip. It hurt much more than the ones they used for blood tests.

"Yes. The same as before."

"I don't think so."

"Okay Jesse. I'll tell him."

He paused a moment, then: "Mom, can I have a bag of chips if I'm good?"

"Yes, I'll buy you a bag of chips."

"Okay, I'll have the needle. I'm tough," he said, flexing his muscles. "I'm an Armstrong."

I called Doctor Matthews immediately, and he started the test shortly afterward. I stayed until it was over. Dr. Matthews said it went well. He thanked me again and told me that he would send me the results if they discovered any new information.

When I arrived the next day, our final day, Jesse was sound asleep, still feeling the effects of the previous evening's sedative. I looked around for his breakfast tray which should have been here long ago. When I inquired at the nursing station, I was told that it had come at seven-thirty, as usual, and Dr. Matthews had helped Jesse eat his breakfast.

Jesse was groggy for most of the morning. I packed his suitcases while he dozed. Francine picked us up after lunch and we went to Old Montreal for a couple of hours before boarding the plane for home.

# 11 / "Bad Mother"

Jesse and Tara began the new school year in grades three and two, respectively. Jesse was to be on a modified program, with special help according to his needs.

Chris and I went to see Dr. Lowry to discuss the protocol for the high-dose steroids Dr. Andermann had recommended. I didn't like it, and told him so. "What do you honestly think?" I asked.

"I haven't seen any reports on the results of this program. I know Dr. Andermann is strongly suggesting you try it. But it's an extremely high dose." Dr. Lowry seemed as concerned as we were. "Jesse would have to be monitored in the hospital and have the drugs administered intravenously for the first while."

"What side effects can we expect?" Chris asked.

"Bloating, weight gain, an excess of hair growth, and possibly stomach upset."

"Would you put your child on this program?"

"I don't know. There is no treatment for this disease other than hemispherectomy, and it's much too early to consider that. Perhaps you should give Dr. Andermann a call and discuss it further."

I reached Dr. Andermann early the following morning. "Have you started the steroid program?" he asked.

"That's what I'm calling about. I need to know more about the results they're getting in France. Do you have any statistics?"

"The results look promising," was all he would say.

That wasn't good enough. I wanted to know exactly what had happened to those kids. "I gather from Dr. Dulac's article, which you gave me to read, that the children had a relapse when the program was discontinued. I'm afraid I fail to see the promise."

His voice rose. "Dr. Dulac is a very careful person. This program is your only hope of stopping the deterioration."

"If you can't tell me anything more positive than what I've read in this paper, then I don't think the program is worth the risk."

"Mrs. Armstrong"—his voice was cold—"I think you're a bad mother for not giving your son this chance."

I lost it.

"What chance?" I demanded. "The chance to develop leukemia and liver damage on top of Rasmussen's? You can't give me *any* positive long-term results from your experiments, yet you expect me to let you use my son as a guinea pig! It's not *my* integrity that's in question, Dr. Andermann!" I slammed down the receiver.

I had heard nothing from the school in the first weeks of the new school year, and assumed that things were under control. We had agreed to work closely and stay in contact. I insisted that I be informed as soon as any problem arose. So when I was summoned to the school for a meeting, I didn't know what to expect. I was certainly not prepared for the principal, a superintendent, and Jesse's teacher, all looking grim.

The superintendent began by telling me that Jesse was not behaving at all well, and he was disturbing other children. The stress on the teacher was approaching an intolerable level. The other children, too, were becoming increasingly impatient with Jesse, and it was only a matter of time before their parents began to call.

"This all happened overnight?" I inquired.

"Well, no. It's been getting worse since school began."

"I thought we were all committed to catching these problems before they began."

"We didn't want to alarm you until we had some alternate plan to suggest. For now, we'd like you to take him out of school until we can come to a more suitable arrangement, one that's more beneficial to Jesse."

"Exactly what is he doing?"

Until now Jesse's teacher had sat by, saying nothing, looking for all the world like a fragile flower bent over by a raindrop. Now she said, her voice small and tentative, "It's hard to keep him on task. At story-time he gets up and walks around. Or he talks while I'm trying to read. Sometimes he pushes the other children and tries to get first in line. He's very demanding. I have twenty-five other students' needs to attend to. The children are starting to complain."

The superintendent stepped into the silence. "Roberta is having a difficult time coping with this situation, and we certainly don't want to lose her. And we have to think of Jesse, too. What if one of the children decides to retaliate? He may get hurt."

"I know Jesse is impulsive," I said, struggling to maintain my composure, "and his attention span is getting shorter. That's because of the brain damage the disease is causing. It's not his fault. But if you want me to take him out of school, then I'll take him out."

"If you'll give us a week or so, I can set up a more suitable arrangement. Possibly we could hire a part-time teacher to work with Jesse one-on-one. Or maybe Jesse could come half days. He does seem less manageable after lunch. Maybe half days are all he can manage. Home schooling is another possibility."

"Fine, I'll take him out at noon."

"Oh, no, you don't have to do that," he protested. "You can let him finish the day."

"I'll take him out at noon," I repeated, and went home and made an appointment with Dr. Quinn to take another look at Ritalin.

Two days later the principal and superintendent came to speak to me about the arrangements they had made for Jesse. The school board had approved the funding to hire a teacher. Jesse would remain in the classroom most of the time, and she would be there to help him. Jesse could return to school the following week.

A few hours after they left, Chris and Jesse and I were in Dr. Quinn's office. Jesse was pale and weak from constant seizures; he had been having them every fifteen minutes.

Dr. Quinn was extremely sympathetic to our situation. He explained the effects of Ritalin again, and assured us that we would see it working within a few days. If we didn't see a change, Jesse could easily be taken off it.

I felt neither grateful nor ungrateful, only defeated.

The religion teacher approached me one day as I was picking Jesse up from school. She said Jesse was having difficulty concentrating, but it was more a problem for Tara than it was for her. When Jesse was misbehaving, Tara tried to reprimand him, as if she felt it was her responsibility to keep him in line. She was embarrassed by his actions. I said I would take Jesse out of catechism and teach him at home. I didn't want to ruin Tara's life in the process of trying to save Jesse's.

I had stressed the importance of family to Tara. I had told her that we would all have to deal with the situation, that she might have to play with Jesse more than another sister would because he might have no one else to play with. She was not to treat him like other kids treated him. Friends might come and go but Jesse truly loved her, and that would never change.

In her child's mind, she had translated my desire that she care about Jesse into caring *for* him. I had to lift that burden from her shoulders.

"But, Mom," she said, almost crying when I broached the matter, "he's always hugging and interrupting and bothering, and his colouring is so bad, and he won't *listen*."

"That's because of what's happening in his brain. He can't help the things he does."

She began to cry then. I was surprised by the suddenness and the violence of it. Then I recalled how I had broken down—suddenly, inconsolably—the day Jesse and I had first come back from Montreal. All her frustrations came pouring out in a rush.

"Why did it have to happen to *him*?"

"I don't know," I said. "But it did happen, and we have to deal with it."

"It's hard for me, too, Mom! Sometimes you yell at me for yelling at Jesse, but sometimes he bugs me and bugs me and I get mad at him and when we're at some place he won't listen to me and he won't quit it and I don't know what to do!"

"I am so sorry you have to go through this, Tara. If you'd tell me what happened right away, then I could deal with it."

"But then you get mad at Jesse and you yell at him. It seems like you're always mad."

"I'm sorry, Tara," I said, again, but how could the words take away the pain she was feeling? "I try to be patient. Sometimes I get angry with him and I yell too much. But I really am trying. I feel badly, too, when I act this way. I know how hard it is for you because it's hard for me and you're just a little girl."

"But why do you yell at him when he forgets?"

"It's wrong, I know. But I think that if I push him or make him do something, then maybe he'll remember the next time."

"But you know he can't remember, so why do you get mad again?"

"For the same reason you get mad when you know he can't help it. It doesn't mean we don't love him."

"I know." Her words were barely audible, she was sobbing so hard. "I luh-luh-love him so much!"

I held her and rocked her in my arms. "I know you do. I love Jesse, too. And it's okay to be angry with him sometimes."

"He always wants to play with me, and I need some time with my friends. It's not 'cause I don't love him, but I need to be alone sometimes."

"I do try to keep that in mind. Dad and I let you go for sleep-overs, or to someone's house to play, or do things on your own, don't we?"

"Yes, but when I'm at home I always have to play with him, or if my friends come over you always say that Jesse can play with us."

"Well, it's hard for Jesse because no one will play with him, and he just wants to play. But if that's how you feel, we'll try to give you more time with your friends."

She was silent for a moment, then she asked, "Mom, do you think we could go out sometimes, just me and you?"

"I guess I don't spend a lot of time with you, do I? It's not because I love Jesse more. It's because he's sick and needs me more right now. Maybe later it will be different. Someday everything will be all right, you'll see."

I held her tightly and rocked her back and forth, but inside I wondered if anything would ever be all right again.

Another meeting at the school, this time to meet the new teacher. She was a young woman and this was her first teaching job. She was soft-spoken and seemed friendly. The school had decided that it was in Jesse's best interests to attend in the mornings only. He was increasingly tired, and they thought the three hours in the morning would be all he could handle. We agreed to give it a try.

I received a letter from Kathy and Brian Usher in Connecticut. They sent me a picture of Beth two years after her hemispherectomy, along with some names and addresses of other families who had children with Rasmussen's. Kathy had sent a videotape of Beth to a family in Colorado who were going to record some scenes of their own child and then send it on to us.

The tape and accompanying letter arrived within days. Beth walked with a limp and had little use of her right arm, but she was alive and running and seizure free. Brandi, the little girl from Colorado, had been four-and-a-half years old when her seizures started. She was now six. The videotape had been made two and a half months post-op. Unlike Beth, she did not have a hemiparesis or any weakness going into surgery, but she was plagued by hundreds of seizures every day. She was still unsteady, but she walked unassisted and seemed to be a happy child. Her parents, Cindy and Steven Binder, were extremely happy with the results. They knew they had made the right decision.

This gave me hope. Here was solid evidence that these children had a future. There was life after Rasmussen's Encephalitis. But it was the timing of the surgery that seemed to be what decided the quality of that life.

Jesse continued to have one or two seizures a day throughout October, not counting the muscle jerks, the arm jerks, the laughing seizures, and the short-pause seizures. His stomach-aches were also frequent. His weight continued to drop and he no longer cared for any kind of meat. He often turned down treats, and he never asked for anything to eat. We continued doing blood tests. Dr. Lowry called at the end of the month with another increase in the anticonvulsants, as the last levels were low. Jesse was now on 2,000 milligrams of Depakene, 1,000 milligrams of Tegretol, and 10 milligrams of Ritalin a day. He was seeing double occasionally, even though his blood levels were within range. He was always sluggish, and it seemed to cost him a great deal of effort even to speak.

Reports from school indicated the Ritalin was keeping him more on task and helping with his attention span. They were trying some behaviour management strategies, and continued to monitor his seizures.

At the end of the month, Jesse and I saw Jo Nanson, a neuro-psychologist at the Alvin Buckwold Centre in Saskatoon. She had done a battery of tests, and concluded that the results of the intelligence tests done in Montreal—that Jesse had suffered no measurable deterioration in comparison with last year—were inconsistent with his early history. She suggested that he had, in fact, experienced a noticeable decline in intellectual skills. She also noted that his behaviour was impulsive and he had trouble listening to directions. He exhibited significant problems in learning new verbal material, and his short-term memory for both verbal and visual material was deteriorating. Because of the myoclonus in both hands, she suggested he be taught to type, as he would likely be incapable of cursive writing.

At the beginning of November, Dr. Lowry wrote a letter to Dr. Freeman at Johns Hopkins, asking him to assess Jesse and give us his opinion on disease management. I called Diana Pillas on the 17th, notifying her of Dr. Lowry's letter. She asked me to write to our Medical Insurance Branch to see if they would cover the medical expenses and to write her a letter about our situation.

*Letter to Diana Pillas at John Hopkins Hospital, November 22nd, 1989*
The school has decided that this week Jesse would go from 9:00–2:15 PM to see how he would manage with the extended hours. The last two days, however, I've had to keep him home because of seizures.

There are a few controversies on the management of this disease that are really eating away at me. I'm afraid of waiting too long to do a hemispherectomy and then finding out that it's too late. Or being told at that point that we could have saved more, if only we'd have done something sooner. I have to know that I have done all I could do, including getting a second opinion. If Dr. Freeman's opinion is the same as I've been told then I will come home, accept the decision, and be somewhat at peace knowing that I've done all I can. But I can't sit here wondering if maybe we are missing the boat. There is too much at stake.

Through the whole of December, Jesse was feeling poorly, as if he were suffering a long and lingering flu. His appetite had decreased drastically and he was steadily losing weight. Last year at this time I had had trouble finding clothes that fit because of his swollen belly. Now I was having the same problem for the opposite reason. I tried to coax him to eat, giving him whatever he wanted, whatever he would agree to try. What he did eat, he often vomited up again.

Christmas came and went. Jesse was pale and thin, but he always managed a smile and a bear-grip hug. Sometimes I'd find him wincing and holding his stomach. On Monday, January 8th, he was once again seeing double. It took him all day to eat one piece of toast, and then he was vomiting again.

I took him to Dr. Lowry the following day. He was so weak he couldn't walk a straight line. He weighed forty-eight pounds. Dr. Lowry was mystified. He asked me to bring him back on Thursday when his colleague, Dr. Bruce, could have a look at him.

I took Jesse home, somewhat relieved, believing that Dr. Lowry was going to get to the bottom of this. We only had to wait two days.

Jesse couldn't wait that long.

The next day I heard him fall in his bedroom. I found him lying facedown on the floor, his little body wracked with sobs. He didn't look as if he'd had a seizure.

"What happened, honey?"

"I fell," he said, between sobs.

"Oh, honey, I'm sorry!" I helped him up and carried him to the couch. "I'm going to call Dr. Lowry right now. Do you think you could eat some toast?"

"No, Mom, I feel like throwing up. I don't want to eat anything."

"This is bloody-well ridiculous," I cursed as I reached for the phone. "This is Mrs. Armstrong. I'd like to speak to Dr. Lowry."

"I'm sorry Mrs. Armstrong, Dr. Lowry is with a patient."

"This is important! I have to speak to him *now*!"

I was angry. I wasn't sure at whom, but I was mad as hell. *He's just a little boy. It's not enough that seizures knock him to the ground, but now the medication, the illness . . . what? What the hell is going on now?*

There was a long pause, then, "Dr. Lowry speaking."

"Jesse can hardly stand up. Just now he fell flat on his face! He can't even walk any more!"

"Bring him in," he said. "I'll admit him this morning."

# 12 / One Crisis to Another

Jesse was admitted to Pædiatric Ward 3200. Dr. Bruce came in for a consultation, as Dr. Lowry had requested. He examined Jesse and ordered tests.

I helped get Jesse ready for the night, encouraged him to have a bath, then helped him get in the tub and washed him. When he lay down to wet his hair I was shocked at how thin he was. His head seemed disproportionately large, and his eyes were huge, with pale grey hollows beneath them. I could clearly see the outline of his jawbone. His collarbones, too, were prominent, and I could count every rib. His stomach was concave, his hip bones jutting out on either side. His legs grew down from his torso like toothpicks. He was as pale as the porcelain tub he was lying in. He looked, in short, a picture of death. I wondered if that's what he was. I wondered if his struggle and his life were all for naught.

"Mom, can I get out now? I'm cold."

His hands and feet had been cold to the touch for months. In the past summer he often sat wrapped in a blanket watching TV while the rest of us wore as little as possible to beat the heat.

I helped him out of the tub and got him ready for bed. I asked for an extra blanket and tucked him in. It reminded me of when he was born. The nurses in the maternity ward had shown us first-time mothers how to wrap our babies tightly in a receiving blanket. They liked the restraint, we were told; it made them feel secure.

"Snug as a bug in a rug," I whispered as I wrapped the hospital blankets around him. Snug as a baby in his mother's arms.

Over the next two days Jesse had blood tests, an abdominal ultrasound, a chest X-ray, an upper gastrointestinal X-ray, a CT scan with contrast, and an EEG. Dr. Lowry and Dr. Bruce examined him again, along with countless residents and interns. Dr. Best, a pædiatric endocrinologist, was also called in. When I pointed out the jumpiness in Jesse's eyes, an eye examination was ordered as well.

As they were ready to inject the dye for the CT scan, Jesse clutched his stomach and turned his head to the left. "He's having a seizure," I said to the technician who was poking around for a vein. He looked up at me. "He should just be a minute," I said. I held Jesse's hands. His left hand cupped and turned inward. In a minute it was over. His body relaxed as he closed his eyes.

"Is he all right?"

"He's fine now. You can go ahead."

The scan showed more atrophy in the right frontal lobe compared to six months earlier. The overlying dura in this area had become more calcified. The remainder of the brain appeared normal.

The ultrasound and X-rays were normal.

His EEG was abnormal, showing right and left epileptic discharges from the frontal temporal areas independently, which again raised the question of whether the seizures were originating from both sides.

On Friday Jesse was feeling somewhat better. The vomiting had ceased, and he began eating small amounts. By the time his eyes were examined, the jumpiness in them had disappeared.

Late Friday afternoon I met Dr. Lowry at the nursing station.

"Do you have a few minutes?" he asked.

"I was just coming to talk to you."

"Why don't we go to another room?"

He pointed to a small room with a desk and chair a few feet away. A chill went up my spine, remembering the last time I'd been invited into a little private room: it was when Dr. Andermann had told me my son had Rasmusssen's Encephalitis. Bad news is reserved for small rooms.

"I don't want to go in there," I said, my voice barely a whisper.

He looked at me strangely. "I think it'll be a little more private."

*That's what I'm afraid of.* But I bit my lip and followed him. He shut the door and sat on the corner of the desk, Jesse's chart in his hand.

"Have a seat," he said, and I sat on the edge of the chair.

"There doesn't seem to be any clear explanation for Jesse's symptoms," he continued. "According to the blood work, his kidneys and liver are functioning well. His medication levels are all within range. Neither Dr. Bruce nor Dr. Best can find any abnormalities."

He only wanted to discuss Jesse's case, not give me bad news. I was limp with relief.

"He can't go on like this." I said.

"I'd like to take him off Ritalin for a while. It's his newest medication. I want to make sure it's not causing the problem."

"I took him off Ritalin for two weeks during the Christmas break," I said. "There was no change. I don't think it's the Ritalin."

"I'd like to be absolutely sure. He won't be going to school like this, so it won't hurt to try again." I agreed. "There may be some brain stem involvement that the EEG's not picking up. I don't know what the literature on Rasmussen's has to say on this."

I did, and it opened up a train of thought I didn't care to follow. I tried to sound confident as I said, "There's one recorded case of a patient dying from brain stem involvement, but that was uncertain."

He nodded. We sat in silent thought. Unless it was indeed the brain stem, we were missing something.

"Could you phone Dr. Andermann and see if he's experienced this with any other patient?" I asked.

He glanced at his watch. "It's too late today, but I could try on Monday. Jesse's been feeling better, hasn't he?"

I nodded. "He hasn't vomited since Thursday, and his eyes have stopped jumping. I've been giving him plenty of fluids. He's even eating again."

"That *is* good news," said Dr. Lowry.

"But this has been going on for most of December. The symptoms come for a few days, then disappear for a few days. Please don't send him home," I pleaded. "Don't give up on him. He can't live like this."

"I won't give up on him," Dr. Lowry promised, "but I think you should take him home on a weekend pass and see how he fares. Bring him back Monday morning. That will give me some time to put the test results together and see what we can come up with. I'll speak with Dr. Bruce and Dr. Best again. Don't worry, I won't discharge him until I know we've done all we can."

He was speaking very gently. I wondered if Jesse was dying, and Dr. Lowry needed the weekend to figure out how to tell me.

I discontinued the Ritalin and Jesse seemed to improve. His stomach cramps were at a minimum, and he was eating again. He was still pale and thin, but he didn't vomit, and he didn't stagger.

I retreated to my room and closed the door. I opened the file I had collected on Rasmussen's and searched the case histories until I found what I was looking for. "Only one patient has died of the disease itself," I read:

> She died of an apparent progression of the disease to the brain stem twenty-two months after onset and eleven months after a frontal and temporal lobectomy had been carried out.

Thus, the disease, although progressive over a period of years, is rarely fatal. Ultimately, the underlying causative agent apparently dies out and the patient's neurologic status becomes stable.

Unfortunately, by that time most patients have sustained significant and permanent neurological deficits.

By Sunday evening Jesse was feeling nauseous again, and I was sick with worry myself. I asked Chris what we were going to do. He was silent for a minute.

"We don't know that it's progressed to the brain stem," he said.

"But what if it has? What are we going to do?"

"We'll wait to see what they say next week. Maybe they'll come up with something."

"You know when he phones Montreal, Andermann will throw the high-dose steroids up in our faces and say *I told you so*. That'll be our only option. I hate it. It's wrong, but we'll have no choice. I don't know what to do any more. Oh Chris, I'm so scared."

"I don't want to put Jesse on steroids, either. Let's just wait till next week and see what they have to say."

I was crying now. "But, what are we going to do?"

"I don't know," he said. It hurt him just to talk about it. He couldn't reach out to comfort me any more than I could comfort him. We were dying inside, and neither of us could ease the other's pain.

Monday morning. Jesse was feeling nauseous again, and dizzy, and unable to eat. His eyes were jumping. He had stomach cramps. With a pillow, an ice cream pail, and a box of tissues on the front seat with us, we dropped Tara off at school and headed for the hospital. Jesse looked pathetic. How could he look reasonably well on Saturday and look like death again on Monday?

We made it to the hospital without incident. I spotted a wheelchair as we entered the main hall. I went to grab it, and heard Jesse vomiting behind me. His coat was covered with it. I cleaned his face and hands with a wad of tissue and swept him into the chair. Pausing only to apologize to the girl at the information desk, I took Jesse to his room, where I stripped his clothing and washed him using a basin and cloth; he was clearly too weak to get into the bathtub.

Dr. Bruce stopped by, but he had no new information. He stressed the importance of keeping up Jesse's fluid intake, especially since he'd been vomiting. There was a danger of dehydration.

Jesse lay in bed for most of the day with cramps. Every half hour I urged him to drink something. By late afternoon the cramps had subsided.

By evening, he was able to eat a little. On Tuesday he was sitting up for most of the day, and eating more. His face showed a bit of colour. We continued to push the fluids.

We saw Dr. Lowry on Wednesday morning. He had been unable to reach Dr. Andermann. He'd read over the literature on Rasmussen's and was unable to come up with anything concrete.

"What do you think?" he asked.

He knew I had read every paper published on Rasmussen's, but this was the first indication that he actually valued my opinion. It meant more to me than I had expected.

"I wonder if he could be toxic on his medicine. He's shown the same effects from toxicity, except these symptoms are intensified."

"We rechecked the blood levels," he said. "They're all within range."

He sat looking at his papers, deep in thought. I sat on the chair, trying to put the last six months together, find some connection, some explanation.

"I've been wondering about Tegretol for a long time," I said. "Whenever he gets to 800 milligrams, his symptoms seem to indicate he's toxic, even though the blood levels are always within the therapeutic range."

He thought for a few moments longer, then something struck him: "You know, I have read about Carbamazepine [Tegretol] epoxide, a metabolic breakdown product which may produce signs of toxicity, and which isn't demonstrable by our usual laboratory test. Maybe that's it. We could try reducing the Tegretol and, if his symptoms don't recur, we could eliminate it and maintain him on Depakene alone."

"It's worth a shot," I said.

Jesse was discharged later that day. Dr. Lowry had set up a schedule to reduce the Tegretol by 100 milligrams every four days while keeping a close eye on the Depakene. The aim was to minimize Jesse's seizures while the Tegretol was being decreased. After ten days, we knew we'd found the answer. Jesse's double vision was gone, along with the vomiting, the staggering, and the stomach cramps. His seizures averaged two a day. He was still thin and pale, but he was out of immediate danger, and he wasn't in constant pain.

Ten days later the seizures returned with a vengeance: five the first two days, ten the next, then twenty-eight. It was January 29th, 1990. Jesse was waking up every twenty minutes with another seizure. Chris slept in Jesse's room while Jesse slept with me. It was a fairly frequent arrangement

All through the night, we kept our vigil. The room was pitch black. I'd be awakened by a whispered, "Mom." I'd reach out to him as the seizure began. I could feel his body wracked with it, until it seemed to enter mine. My words were almost invariable: "It's okay, Honey. It'll be done soon. It's okay, Jesse." I could feel the energy draining out of him. Then a short exhalation, his body relaxed, and we both fell into a deep sleep. Every twenty minutes the ritual was repeated.

I barely heard the alarm ring at 7:30. Yet, if it had whispered, "Mom," I would have been wide awake instantly. I staggered through to the kitchen and made breakfast.

"What's wrong?" Tara asked.

"Jesse had seizures all night."

"Oh," was her only response. She was used to it.

Jesse was settled on the couch. I asked her to check on him. She called back, "He's having a seizure."

"Stay with him till he's done, Tara. I have to make your lunch."

I could hear her talking to him: "It's okay Jesse. It's okay. It'll be done soon." I knew she was holding his hands. I'd seen her do it many times. She had learned it from me. The only reason I didn't scream out, *This isn't right! This isn't normal! This should not be a ritual!* is that I was too numb.

I placed a cold face-cloth on his forehead for the headache, and gave him an Ativan for the seizures. Then I called Dr. Lowry. We had expected an increase in seizures since we started reducing the Tegretol. But this was too much. Back to the hospital we went. Dr. Lowry decided to put him on telemetry, as it seemed an opportune moment to record some seizures. In two hours they recorded five.

Jesse was exhausted. He hadn't eaten since early yesterday, and he was too ill to eat yet. We walked slowly back to Dr. Lowry's office, where Doris Newmeyer was waiting for us, cheerful as ever. "Dr. Lowry said to start an IV of Dilantin. Let's bring him in and lay him down."

She felt for a vein.

"Better use the right arm," I said, "The needle may come out in a seizure on the left."

The needle found it's river first try. *Thank God for small mercies,* I thought. Then Jesse clutched his stomach and went into another seizure. His left arm started to jerk, and he almost sat up with the violence of it. We stood by to hold him down in case he went into convulsions. But it was over soon. His eyes rolled back and he fell asleep. The Dilantin flowed through his veins and held the seizures at bay.

I watched him as he slept, and wondered where this was all going. One crisis to another. Was this one over? When would the next one begin? And Lord, when would it all end?

For the rest of February, Jesse averaged one or two seizures a day. He continued to have stomach-aches and arm-jerks. He almost always fell asleep after a seizure. Some days he slept more than he was awake.

Not unnaturally, I was deeply depressed. I felt I was losing him. I was afraid of the future even as I anxiously awaited word from Johns Hopkins.

On March 18th I spoke to Diana Pillas on the telephone. She told me that Dr. Freeman had received copies of Jesse's test results from Dr. Andermann's office, at Dr. Lowry's request, but he needed the biopsy slides as well as copies of the MRIs, not just reports on them. Assuming she received these items soon, she anticipated an April admission.

I called Montreal and managed to get that particular ball rolling. I called the Kinsmen Foundation, who said—bless them—that we had already been approved for funding. I had only to call the travel agent when I had an admission date.

On March 22nd and 23rd Jesse had forty seizures, then none for three days. On March 27th the call finally came from Johns Hopkins. We were to fly to Baltimore on April 2nd and be admitted on the 3rd for a week's stay.

# 13 / Johns Hopkins

We spent our first night in Baltimore at Ronald McDonald House. After the long, worrisome plane trip it was a relief to be in a spacious, clean, comfortable place where I could relax after a tense day of keeping watch over Jesse.

At 9:00 the next morning Jesse was admitted to Johns Hopkins Hospital and brought to physio- and occupational therapy, where they videotaped him to assess his gross and fine motor movement. We were told he would be having an MRI much later in the evening, but I could sleep on a cot by his bed. "Much later" turned out to be 1:30 AM.

Jesse and I were in the playroom the next day after lunch when Dr. Freeman came in. Tall and lanky, and with a warm smile, he greeted us both and asked us how our trip had been. Then he listened until I had answered completely.

Jesse pretty much ignored us, roaming the room looking for something interesting to play with. He knew the routine. Doctors didn't often acknowledge his presence. They usually asked me the questions. But Dr. Freeman spoke directly to Jesse, as if he was important as a person and not just an interesting case. This was new to me, and I had to bite my tongue to keep from answering for him as I usually did. Dr. Freeman had treated fourteen other Rasmussen's patients, but he had a way of making us feel we were more than just the next in line.

He spoke of early hemispherectomy and told us he had seen many children regain intellectual function after surgery. The success rate was based on many factors, including the age of the patient and the amount of deterioration he or she had suffered at the time of surgery.

"I've reviewed the biopsy slides and the other test results," he said. "While some patients have fewer symptoms of the disease and others more, Jesse's pathology reveals most of the features encountered in this syndrome. There's no question in my mind that this is indeed Rasmussen's Encephalitis."

Hearing the diagnosis confirmed brought us a step closer to a successful treatment, or so it seemed to me.

"What now?" I asked.

"Tomorrow Jesse will be moved to our electro-encephalograph monitoring unit. He'll be there for a few days so we can record his seizures. Once I've reviewed the results I'll give you my assessment."

Before he left, he asked me to write an inventory of Jesse's deterioration to give him a clearer picture of what he was like now compared to what he had been like before the onset of the disease. Jesse was then taken to neuropsychology to assess his impulsiveness.

I finally met Diana Pillas, who had been so helpful over the telephone. Her face matched her voice: attractive, confident, and reassuring. She showed me photographs of their Rasmussen's patients—"our kids," she called them—and spoke of the positive results of hemispherectomy. She was straightforward about the possible complications, too, and encouraged me to ask questions of her or Dr. Freeman at any time during our stay.

*Inventory of Jesse's deterioration for Dr. Freeman, April 5th, 1990*

My boy is gone, but he's right here, physically, in someone I don't recognize as my own. He reminds me every day that he is here, and yet he is not.

By grade one, Jesse seemed to be distracted a lot of the time. He had no inhibitions and very few emotions. I tried to ignore his quirks, or talk myself out of their existence. I was so successful at it that I was genuinely surprised when his teacher told us that Jesse was acting strangely. He was changing. He got steadily worse in grade two and three.

Jesse seems to see all of the background and none of the foreground. While you're talking to him he will suddenly wave at a child going by outside, or pick up a pencil and start tapping it. If you take the pencil away, he wants it back, and when you continue talking to him his eyes keep darting toward the pencil. If there is any other distraction, it will claim his attention, displacing anyone who is speaking to him. He may walk away in the middle of a sentence to look at something he has focused on. I'm sure he can't help himself. I know it, in fact, but sometimes I can't help getting upset with him anyway.

In everything, he seems obsessed with what he wants to do, and nobody else matters. This may have to do with his lack of emotions.

He has lost the facility for planning or forethought. He never thinks of consequences. He sees, he wants, he does.

No matter how many times he has been told not to do something, and told the reasons why he shouldn't do it, and even when he has agreed never to do it again, the next time he wants to do it, he does it. "Don't jump on people. Don't grab them and hug them if they don't want to be hugged. Don't keep touching people as you talk to them; your friends don't like it." It's obvious they don't like it, but Jesse has lost the art of reading other people's expressions. He will interrupt anyone, anywhere, at any time if he wants to say something.

He has to tidy his room over and over again. He always leaves things on the floor. He plays on the floor with one toy and leaves it there when he grabs something else. He goes for whatever he wants and forgets about the previous toy, so it stays where it was last used. Over and over we tell him he has to put the previous thing away before he goes on to the next, and he agrees, but he doesn't do it, and then it's, "Oh yeah, I forgot."

He tells me proudly that he's cleaned his room, and brings me to see it, expecting praise. But each time he's picked up one or two things, and left the other twenty where they lay. Then he gets upset when I tell him it's not done properly. Jesse craves approval constantly.

He never listens the first time you tell him something. While we're watching TV, for example, he'll start humming or tapping his fingers. You ask him to stop and he says "'kay," then a few seconds later, or sometimes immediately, he starts again. So you tell him to stop, and he says "'kay" again, and starts again. We've tried ignoring it, but he persists till it drives you crazy and you have to shout, "Quit it!"

I sometimes send him to his room, but I have to tell him at least twice before he'll go, then all the way down the hall he keeps stopping and saying, "I won't do it again," and he keeps saying it until I say, "Go to your room! Go!" and he keeps saying, "I won't do it again," all the way to his room. This happens virtually every time he is in the living room with us and there isn't a cartoon on TV. It also happens when he sits on you, or pokes you and touches you and strokes you. You ask him to push over or stop it, and he says "'kay" and keeps on doing it.

Sometimes you think he's doing it just to drive you crazy. You can scream at him and yell and have a fit and cry, and it just doesn't register. Seconds later, he'll ask you to play cards with him. You may feel like strangling him, but he can't read your expression. This is the main reason he doesn't have friends any more—that and his lack of imagination. His imagination has deteriorated steadily, so that he can no longer contribute to play activities like other children.

He takes everything literally. He doesn't understand when someone is joking with him, especially if they're being sarcastic. He will laugh, but only after they do, or only after they explain themselves. Then, whether or not he gets it, he over-reacts. He'll laugh uproariously at some simple joke, a cartoon, or something trivial that would normally produce no more than a smile. If he makes a joke himself, or says something funny, he'll keep repeating it, over and over. He doesn't realize that a joke isn't that funny the second or third or tenth time around. So I don't encourage laughter with Jesse, because the result is usually less than funny.

If he over-reacts to humour, though, he seems indifferent to people's feelings and emotions. His response to human suffering is mechanical. He has been taught how he should feel, but he can't feel it.

The term "disinhibited anti-social behaviour," unfortunately, describes him well. It doesn't bother him to pick his nose in public, or to hold his penis through his pants. It doesn't seem to embarrass him, and he keeps on doing it no matter how many times he is told to stop.

His verbal skills have also deteriorated. He finds it difficult to express himself. When he's relating a story or an idea, he usually begins somewhere in the middle. He never says who he's talking about, where it happened, what it is they did. A mild example of this occurred a few minutes ago. He said to me, "I like it when they do that."

"When who does what?" I asked.

"I like it when Dads tell their babies to smile for the camera."

Usually it takes him a few more tries, with more prompting from the listener, to get the idea out. Even then, it's often unclear. And most of the time we have no idea what prompted him to speak in the first place. It usually has nothing to do with the current or even the previous conversation.

I don't understand him. I don't know him. I don't recognize him. Worse than that, I don't like him as much as I liked my Jesse before. I know he needs my love as much as he ever did, and I do feel that I sometimes fail him. I feel badly for him. I feel badly for me, too.

When you give Jesse an inch, he takes a mile, so that we've had to cut down on the inches. I can't just give him a hug or a kiss or say, "I love you." If I do, he grabs me around the neck and hugs me until it hurts and he kisses and kisses until I'm disgusted by his behaviour, but if I tell him, "Okay, Jesse, that's enough," it doesn't mean anything to him. He won't stop until I get upset and force him to stop.

Consequently, I don't initiate these moments nearly as often as I used to.

If I say to my daughter, "Tara, you're so cute," or, "Tara, you're being silly today," she'll wave a hand dismissively and say, "Oh, Mom," which is fine and funny. But poor Jesse doesn't know when to quit. If you say something endearing to Jesse, he won't just wave a hand dismissively. He'll push you, or put his fists up, or grab you and squeeze—all of which can be a childish reaction to make it funny, but he always pushes too hard and too long, and he never quits when you've had enough. We may be laughing at first, but it usually goes on too long and we end up being upset.

Jesse has trouble with visual memories and perceptions. For example, I'll have to explain what hamburgers look like before he'll remember what the word "hamburger" means. Another kind of example is when he'll say that he thinks this is Uncle Ernie driving up because he sees a large silver car, when in fact Uncle Ernie drives a small grey Toyota. He'll say that someone looks exactly like Tara when the only resemblance is the length of her hair.

This distorted perspective is apparent in his drawings, too, where boy, girl, mother, and father all look alike, except that sometimes he puts longer hair on the girls. His pigs, dogs, cats, and horses are all constructed the same way. It's hard to understand how two people can look at the same thing yet see different things. Maybe healthy eyes are for healthy vision, but you need a healthy brain to interpret that vision.

Jesse was hooked up to telemetry for five days. The electro-encephalo-gram monitoring unit consisted of four private rooms, each with a bed with side rails, and a bathroom with toilet, tub, and sink. The rooms were large and bright, with a window taking up over half of one wall. There was a television in each room, and a monitor that showed what the overhead camera was filming. The camera itself hung from the ceiling on a pivot. Everywhere Jesse moved, the camera followed. It was spooky at first. It took a while to get used to it.

The rooms were monitored twenty-four hours a day, usually by a single nurse. It was her job to change the videotapes as they filled up. Hers was also the invisible hand moving the camera. There was an intercom in each room so she could communicate with the patient. Most of the time, she just watched and listened. When she saw a seizure developing, she alerted the nursing staff to the appropriate room.

The first two days were extremely long. Jesse was hooked up to the

EEG and couldn't leave the room, so I stayed with him almost constantly. We played games over and over. When I saw a seizure developing, I pressed a button to mark the spot on the tape. At first, Jesse had plenty of arm jerks and short absences, but they were over by the time I got to the button. I was worried that I wasn't catching them, but the nurse reassured me that the machine automatically marked the tape five minutes prior to when the button was pushed. By the end of the first day they had recorded enough of these smaller seizures, and asked me to mark only the stronger ones from then on.

As Jesse's dosage of anticonvulsants was reduced, his absence seizures became stronger. After the first one, the nurse came on the speaker: "Mrs. Armstrong, could you move aside when Jesse is having a seizure? You're blocking the camera."

"I'll try to stay out of the way," I said. "But I've always held his hands while he's in a seizure."

After two more strong absences, the voice interrupted again: "Mrs. Armstrong, I'm afraid you're still getting in the way. Perhaps it's best if you don't touch him at all."

I agreed, though it felt wrong to stand by and do nothing. When he went into a *grande mal* I knew it was important that it be recorded clearly. I watched him twisting on the bed, his facial muscles tightening, his hand jerking inward. *If I could just straighten out his body,* I thought, *put a pillow under his head.* I grabbed a pillow and stuffed it between the bed and the side rails, then stepped back and watched helplessly as the electrical storm spread and the convulsions began. He fell back, his arms, legs, and head jerking uncontrollably. All I could do was stand aside and reassure him with my voice. I felt I was abandoning him. I could almost hear his frantic thoughts—*Mom? Where are you, Mom?* It was small consolation to hear the nurse say, "That's good Mrs. Armstrong. I'm getting a clear shot now."

Each day he had more seizures. His stomach-aches became frequent, and most of his meals were returned untouched. Each night I opened the cot and positioned it next to Jesse's bed. A red light bathed the room in a dim red glow. It was enough light for the camera, should he have a seizure in the night. By the fourth night, he was being awakened by them, and all I could do was call to him from my cot.

Dr. Freeman came every day. On Monday he came early, pulled up a chair, and asked me to sit down. Jesse was sleeping.

"We're recording some good seizures," he told me. "I'll have to examine the EEG recordings and tapes more closely, but from what I've been told it seems that all his seizures are originating from the right hemisphere, mostly from the frontal temporal area."

"So you don't think any are originating from the left hemisphere?" At long last I was able to set that particular worry aside.

"No, I don't think so. The frequent seizures are likely interfering with the left hemisphere. That's another reason I believe in early hemispherectomy. The sooner we can remove the diseased hemisphere, the less interference it will create with the healthy one, and the more chance there is for intellectual growth."

"Do you think it's time for a hemispherectomy?"

"What do you think?" he countered. "Are *you* ready for this surgery?"

It was a tough question. It would be easier to wait until the disease gave us no other choice, but could I honestly say that waiting was in Jesse's best interest? What if it took another five years before he showed signs of hemiparesis? Assuming he didn't go into status and die in the interim, he would certainly have deteriorated, intellectually and socially, a great deal more than he had already. He would have been in and out of hospital, suffered thousands of seizures, not to mention stomach pains, nausea, and vomiting. It might be easier to operate when Jesse had nothing left to lose, but would there be any hope of regaining anything by then?

On the other hand, was I prepared to remove half my son's brain, deliberately depriving him of the use of his left hand and leg, if it wasn't yet necessary? And what about all the other functions I didn't know about, the ones I couldn't see or evaluate? If he truly was in the early stages of the disease, he could be physically whole for years yet.

I said to Dr. Freeman, "I honestly don't know if I could go through with it."

"How does your husband feel about it?"

"He worries about Jesse, but I don't think he sees the deterioration as much I do. I don't know how he feels about surgery. We don't talk about it much. What do you recommend?"

"This is a difficult one to call. Jesse is obviously having frequent seizures, but they're not yet as frequent as they can be with Rasmussen's. He doesn't have any contra-lateral weakness, and his motor area is not yet involved. Against that we have to balance the long-term effects of the interference with his left-frontal lobe and intellect, and we have to be aware of how much he stands to regain once the right hemisphere is removed. Taking that and your own feelings into account, I suggest you keep early hemispherectomy in mind, but wait for some evidence of a left hemiparesis, a more rapid intellectual deterioration, or an increase in seizures. I believe all of these will come."

He told us we could go home on Wednesday.

The following day, Jesse was disconnected from the EEG. He was still having frequent seizures, even though they had renewed his medication. By the end of the day he hadn't eaten anything, and was worn out from the battering of the disease. His stomach-aches were constant and he didn't want to get out of bed. I asked the nurse if they could give him something to stop the seizures. They gave him an Ativan.

The following day, Jesse and I flew to Toronto. On the flight, I asked him what he would do if we told him they could take away his seizures but he would have to give up using his left arm. "Do you think that would be worth it?"

"So, I would just have one arm? You mean, forever?"

"Yes, but your seizures would be gone."

He thought a moment. "I don't think so, Mom. I need two hands to do stuff."

"Okay."

The decision was easier now I knew where Jesse stood. He was sick much of the time, but I don't know if he was able to relate his illness to the seizures. He didn't remember most of them. In themselves, then, the seizures didn't bother him much.

Chris's mother met us at the airport and drove us through Toronto to Richmond Hill. Off in the distance you could see "Wonderland," with it's radiant lights flashing.

*Some day,* I thought, as I had many times before, *some day when this is all over, I'll take Jesse to Disneyland.*

We had a nice visit with Chris's family, and flew home the following morning.

# 14 / The End of My Rope

When I received the results of the neuro-psychological testing in Baltimore, I was shocked. Jesse's IQ appeared to have dropped drastically in the past year. I knew he was declining mentally, but previous tests had always indicated the deterioration was marginal. I immediately called Jo Nanson, Jesse's neuro-psychologist at the Alvin Buckwold Centre in Saskatoon, and asked her if the Baltimore WISC tests were based on the same standards as the ones she used. She assumed they were, but said she would call Johns Hopkins to make sure.

Jesse's impulsiveness had reached new heights, and his behaviour was now a constant annoyance to everyone around him. He couldn't watch TV for any length of time unless it was a cartoon. And if Jesse wasn't watching television, neither could anyone else. He was constantly interrupting or making noises. The same was true about visiting. He made conversation difficult, if not impossible. In the meantime, the seizures varied from one to five a day. He was beginning to vomit again, and lose more weight.

Depression was beginning to overwhelm me. As much as I tried to pull myself out of it, sometimes I just couldn't manage. Most mornings I lay in bed, wishing for the night to return, wishing I could sleep and not have to face the day. I didn't want to see anyone. I didn't want to talk to anyone. At times it took all my energy just to speak. I kept the blinds closed and wished I could stop the phone from ringing. I cried easily and often, mostly at trivial things.

One Saturday the kids and I went to Henriette's house for the week-end. I reminded Jesse, as I always did, not to jump on his cousins, and not to hug them too hard. As always, he agreed. As always, he forgot as soon as he walked in the door. He grabbed my sister and her three children in turn and hugged them until he was told, and told again, to let go. It was his customary greeting. It was also a naked and embarrassing reminder of his immaturity and impulsiveness.

This was an especially trying weekend. I don't know if it was because Jesse behaved worse than usual or if my emotions were running higher than usual, and my depression lower. The breaking point came on the last day when Jesse asked for an apple. Minutes later, he went into the bathroom and came out without it. I realized he had probably thrown it in the garbage. He had little appetite these days and we didn't force him to eat, but when he asked for food we expected him to finish it. He had lied to me before about spitting out food and I had spanked him, making it clear that the punishment was for lying, not for spitting out the food. Lying I would not tolerate. I needed to be able to trust him. I was unsure of almost everything else. If I could not be sure that what he said to me was the truth, I felt there would be nothing left.

"Jesse," I asked, "where is your apple?"

*Please don't tell me you ate it. Don't lie to me.*

"I ate it," he said, avoiding my eyes.

"You couldn't have eaten it that quickly," I said. I got up to check the bathroom, but gave him one last chance. "What did you do with your apple?"

*Tell me now. It's not too late.*

"I ate it, Mom."

I checked the bathroom. The apple was in the garbage.

"You didn't eat it, you pitched it out! Why did you do that?"

"I don't know." He still wasn't looking at me.

I could feel the anger boiling up inside. "Why did you lie to me?" I demanded.

"I don't know." It was his usual answer.

Hen and her kids were silent. Tara was silent. She knew what was coming.

I grabbed Jesse by the shirt and pulled him up the stairs. "You don't know! You don't know!" I was yelling at him. "You *never* know why you do something, you just do it! Why did you throw out the apple?"

"I don't—"

I didn't give him time to say it again. "Why did you lie to me?"

"I don't—"

"You don't know! You don't know! Well, you're going to know better next time, believe me!"

The adrenalin was pumping. I was not going to let him lie to me again. I threw him onto the bed. He was crying, and his eyes were fearful. He was afraid of me, afraid of his own mother. I couldn't control my rage. I didn't try. My hands were shaking as I turned him over and started to spank him.

"Mom, I won't do it again!"

I didn't hear him. I kept spanking him, and I was practically screaming now, "You *don't* lie to me! Don't you ever, *ever* lie to me again!"

"I'm sorry!" he sobbed, as I continued spanking him. I'd lost it. All the fears, the pain, the craziness, the disappointments, the despair: they all came out in that moment, in the rise and fall of my hand on his little bottom.

When it was over, finally, I was drained, devoid of any emotion.

"Stop," I whispered. "Stop this nightmare. Let me get off. I can't take it any more."

I went to bed early when we got home. When Chris crawled in beside me, I whispered, "What are we going to do, Chris?"

"What's wrong?" he asked.

"I can't manage any more. I hurt Jesse." The tears welled up in my eyes. "I hurt my baby. He was scared of me, Chris. I saw it in his face." I began to cry. "I'm no good for him. It's not his fault. God, what am I going to do? I'm losing it."

Chris reached out. I came into his arms, and he held me protectively as I sobbed.

"What am I going to do?" I moaned. "I can't manage any more. I've tried but I can't. I'm doing him more harm than good. I don't want to hurt my boy. What am I going to do?"

"It'll be okay," he said, trying to soothe me.

"No," I said, "it's getting worse and I don't know what to do. When will it end?"

"I don't know," he whispered. "I just don't know."

I cried off and on for the rest of the night, tossing and turning, falling asleep only to wake up and burst into tears again. I felt helpless, in despair. But I finally came to a conclusion: in order to save Jesse, I had to save myself. If I were to crumble, Jesse would surely be lost.

The next day I sat on the examining table in my doctor's office. I had spoken to her once before about my depression, and she had suggested a course of antidepressants. I had flatly refused. I believed, at the time, that we all had control over our emotions, and it was a sign of weakness if we had to depend on drugs to keep them in check. *I'll just have to pull up my socks and take control,* I told myself. But today my socks were hanging very low. I despised the weakness that was making me ask for artificial inner strength, for self-control, self-discipline, and will-power, but I had run out of all three. Could I please buy some at the drug store?

The door opened. "What can I do for you today?" Dr. Wilson asked.

I took a deep breath, trying to hold back the tears. But it was no use. My tear ducts seemed to be connected to my voice box. As soon as I opened my mouth, the dam broke.

"I need some help," I said, or tried to say as the tears streamed down my face. "I can't manage any more. I thought I could do it on my own but I can't."

"You know, Nicky," she said, reassuringly, "there's no shame in needing a bit of help when things are very hard for a very long time. I'm surprised you hung on this long. We'll start with a low dose of a mild antidepressant. What it will do is level out the peaks and valleys, keep you on a more even keel. You don't have to worry about becoming addicted. You can stop taking them at any time."

She wrote me a prescription. I thought I was giving up control when I accepted those pills, but the truth was I had lost it long ago. I was giving up nothing. My control now sat in a child-proof bottle on a shelf beside Jesse's anticonvulsants, another weapon in the arsenal as we struggled to keep the thief at bay.

By the middle of May Jesse was feeling poorly again, with stomach-aches and frequent vomiting. One day his teacher called, asking me to come and get him from school.

"Did he have a seizure?"

"No, he feels sick to his stomach. I think he may have the flu."

"I'll be right there," I said.

I hoped it was the flu. The flu would go away.

I brought him home and tucked him snugly into bed. He fell asleep. When he awakened, I gave him his medicine, but he promptly brought it back up. Dr. Lowry said to bring him in for a blood test.

Jesse looked pale and weak for the next few days, but he wanted to go to school so I let him. Again, his teacher called. Jesse was vomiting in school. Again I brought him home. He looked dreadful. I still hoped it was the flu, but there were no other symptoms, and he was still having seizures.

"How are you feeling today, Honey-bear?"

"Not too good." His face was pale. "I feel like throwing up."

I settled him on the couch with a blanket and pillow. He was feeling dizzy. I brought him a bowl and a box of tissues. A few minutes later he started to vomit.

At 11:30 he was able to eat half a piece of toast and a swallow of water. At 2:00 it all came back up. I called Dr. Lowry again, and he said to reduce the dosage of Dilantin. The blood level results weren't back yet, but he would call me if they were low.

Jesse fell asleep at 4:30. I woke him up at 6:00 to see if he could eat a bit of supper. He said he couldn't. I asked him to try, just a little bit. "Come sit at the table with us and see how it goes."

He walked slowly to the table, his hand on his stomach, and sat there, looking like death. He wanted to eat, but couldn't. He asked if he could go to bed.

"Can't you eat just a little bit, Jess?"

"No, I can't."

"Okay, you go to bed."

He slept through the night, waking up once to have his medicine.

The following day I took him to see Dr. Lowry. The reduced dosage of Dilantin should have helped by now, I reasoned. Dr. Lowry said the last blood level was high. He wanted to do another, to see if the reduction of Dilantin had had any effect. He would call me with the results as soon as he got them.

He called on Friday. The Dilantin was still high. I was to reduce it by a further twenty-five milligrams.

Jo Nanson called shortly afterwards. She had spoken to Johns Hopkins; their tests were the same and the results were valid.

"That's terrible," I said. "What are we going to do?"

"It is a drastic deterioration in one year," Jo said, "but I think we should hang on. We'll retest him in six months."

In the two months since we had returned from Baltimore, I had thought a great deal about hemispherectomy. It seemed to me that the encephalitic brain was like two buns in a bag—one fresh, the other with a spot of mould. As time goes on, the mould spreads, less and less of the bun is useable, and eventually the other one is tainted as well. But at what point do you throw out the mouldy bun? I was afraid of waiting too long. Intellectually and emotionally, the essence of Jesse was dying, but physically he was not dying fast enough for us to save the essence of what he really was.

"Maybe we're wrong to wait for physical deterioration," I said. "He's dying in front of my eyes. How can I watch him become almost non-existent mentally while we wait for him to deteriorate physically so that we won't be creating a deficit?"

"The decrease is severe," Jo allowed, "but I think Jesse would still have a lot more to lose intellectually should you remove that hemisphere now."

I had to agree: it was much easier to justify throwing out a bun once it was covered in mould. Until then, though, how do you justify taking away half a starving man's food supply while claiming that you're trying to keep him alive?

"I really think you should wait six months and retest," she repeated.

Reluctantly, I agreed.

Two days later, the vomiting stopped. But with the Dilantin reduced, he had a *grande mal* on May 28th, another a week later, and another on June 8th. After each episode, his left side was paralysed for ten minutes. In between the *grande mals* he had his regular daily seizures, and would fall asleep after most of them as well.

Softball season was under way, and again we enrolled Jesse. This year, however, the gap between him and the other players in terms of ability had widened. He was becoming disabled in many aspects of his life. Socially he was becoming more immature. Physically he was weakening, and becoming more awkward. Intellectually, he was still losing ground.

We drove to nearby towns for the ball games, never knowing if we would be there the whole time. Jesse usually made it through, but sometimes we would get there only to witness a seizure and then watch him sleep. We'd turn around and come back home.

The antidepressants were working, though. I felt much calmer. My emotions were more even. I didn't plummet to the depths of depression that I had before. I was less confused, and the thoughts that had once raced along were now doing a comfortable jog. Life no longer overpowered me. I began to think I might even survive and not destroy my children in the process.

As strength returned, I felt a renewed determination to save Jesse.

OPPOSITE TOP
*Jesse at three months.*

OPPOSITE BOTTOM
*September 1986: Tara's first day at playschool.*
*This is just before Jesse got sick.*

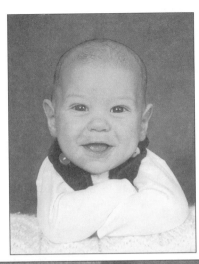

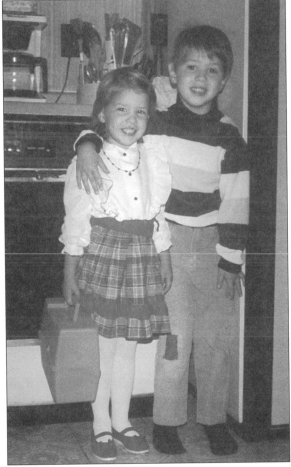

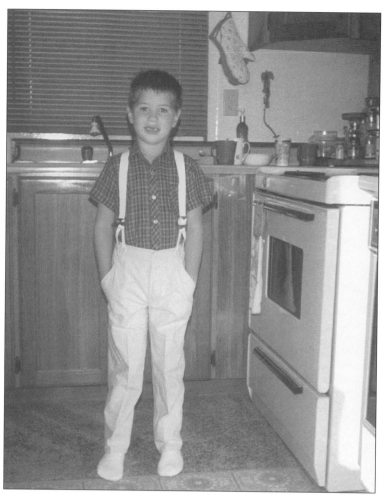

*August 1987. First day of Grade One.*

OPPOSITE TOP
*September 1987. Jesse broke his wrist at school.*

OPPOSITE BOTTOM
*June 1988. Sleeping after a seizure.*

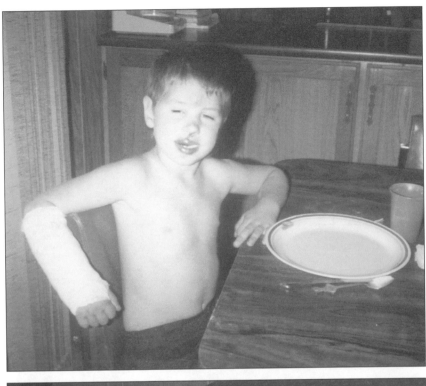

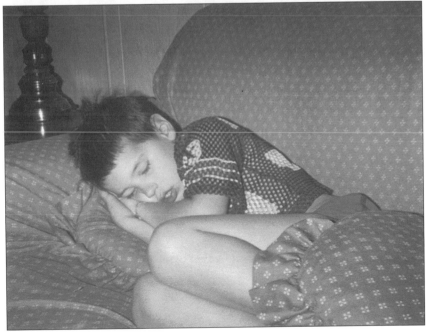

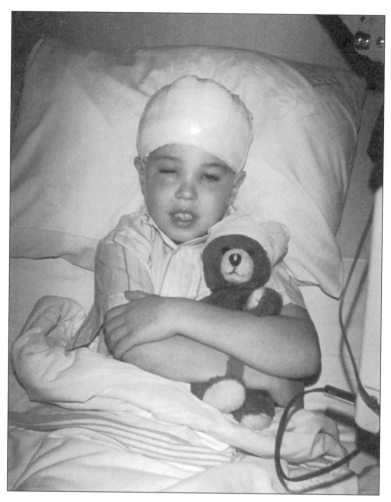

*July 1988. A few days after surgery in Montreal.*

OPPOSITE TOP
*Christmas Eve, 1989. Three years after he first became ill,*
*Jesse was thin and pale, and always had a stomache-ache.*

OPPOSITE BOTTOM
*April 1990. First Communion.*

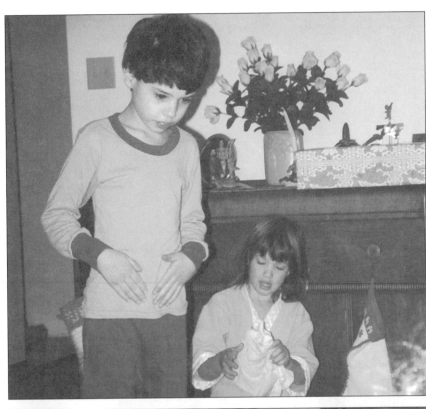

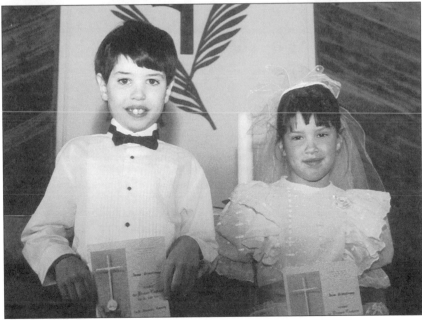

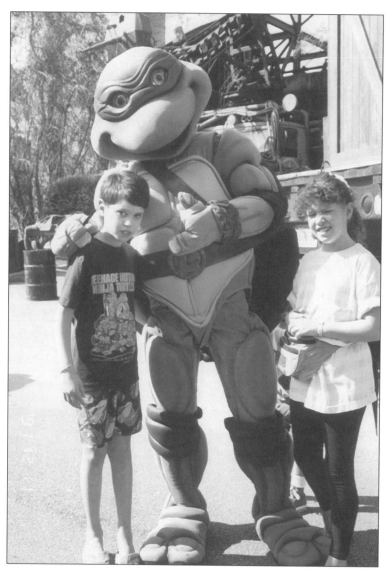

*December 1991. Jesse, Tara, and friend at Disneyland,*
*a month before Jesse's hemispherectomy.*

OPPOSITE TOP
*A week after the hemispherectomy.*

OPPOSITE BOTTOM
*Ten weeks after the hemispherectomy: leaving the hospital.*

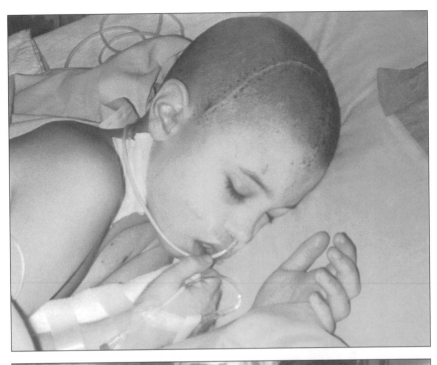

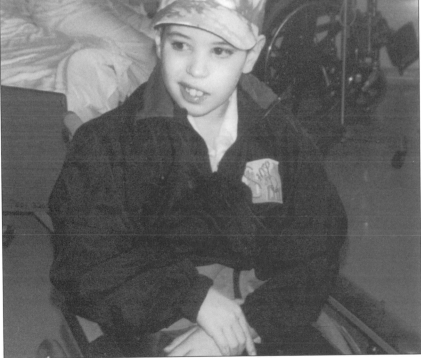

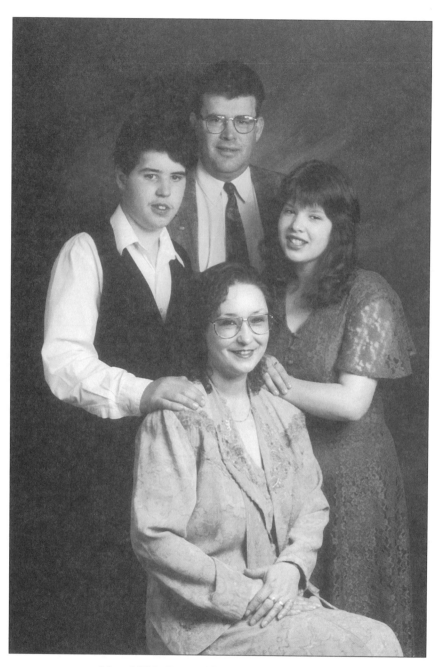

*May 1996. Jesse, Chris, Nicky, and Tara.*

# 15 / On the Same Side, At Last

June arrived, the sun was shining. It should have been a wonderful time. Instead, things seemed to stay bad or get worse. Jesse had five *grande mals* in June, aside from the sixty other seizures he suffered that month. In order to keep track in my diary, I redefined what a seizure was and only recorded those that lasted thirty seconds or longer. I stopped counting the arm jerks, the inexplicable laughter, the stomach cramps, and the times he stopped for a few seconds then "shook it out."

These latter were happening more and more often. His teacher wondered if he might be doing it for attention. I tried to keep an open mind on all such inquiries or suggestions. Jesse's personality had changed, and I could no longer be sure of anything. But I seriously doubted his "shaking out" seizures were a bid for attention. Surely he had enough real seizures without having to fake any more. Even so, I said I'd keep an eye on him and check with the doctor.

As far as I could tell, Jesse had the seizures whether we were with him or not, whether he was outside or in his room, whether he knew I was watching him or not. He would shake them out and continue what he was doing. I tried ignoring him while he was having one. He didn't mind, but Tara found it difficult.

"Mom, Jesse's having a seizure."

"I know."

"Aren't you going to go to him?"

"He'll be fine."

Nothing we did changed the nature or frequency of the seizures. They neither increased when we acknowledged them, nor decreased when we ignored them. Dr. Lowry agreed they were probably another type of seizure. I told Jesse's teacher that the neurologist and I both believed

Jesse's "shaking out" episodes were indeed small seizures.

On June 17th another new type of seizure appeared. I was watching Jesse and Tara playing basketball on the patio when suddenly his arms dropped to his sides and he slumped forward. Then he straightened up again.

"Jesse, what happened?"

"Seizure," he said, and continued playing.

As odd as these new seizures were, we soon got used to them. It was the severe seizures that were disruptive. Most days he had at least one. He would try hard to stay awake afterwards, especially on the rare occasions when he had a friend over, but usually the friend went home because Jesse had fallen asleep.

It was also in June that some of the seizures increased in intensity. I remember the first one in particular. His whole body tensed as his left hand and foot stiffened and turned inward. Then he began to shake. I had never seen such physical intensity. When it was over he looked utterly drained.

He had two more before supper—neither of which I witnessed, but that wasn't uncommon any more. The second he told me about, because his stomach was sore and he didn't think he could eat. I told him to take a shower and see how he felt then. He wasn't allowed to bathe alone, but showers were safe enough. I always timed them, and if the water ran for more than a few minutes I would check on him. I could tell he'd had a third seizure when he came up. He wouldn't have had time to recover from the paralysis of a *grande mal*, but he looked absolutely wrung out. He asked if he could go to bed. It was only 6:00 o'clock. I hated him going to bed so early, especially on an empty stomach. He was sleeping his life away.

I compromised: "Why don't you lie down on the couch for a while?"

"Okay."

He fell asleep almost immediately. I woke him up at 8:00 to give him his medication, then he was asleep for the night. Many evenings now we talked, ate, watched TV, and lived our lives without Jesse, for he was sleeping after a seizure.

I used to keep him home for the day when he had a seizure before school. But now he was seizing every day. Many mornings I drove him the three blocks to school so I wouldn't worry about him. He was so tired and weak most of the time that he welcomed the ride. He weighed forty-eight pounds.

July was much the same as June: ninety absence seizures and one *grande mal*. He was living mostly on toast with Cheese Whiz. He could tolerate no meat, and we learned not to force the issue. He gagged on most other foods.

Life had to go on. I enrolled him in swimming lessons. He had earned his yellow and orange badges when he was five, but he hadn't taken any lessons since. Four years later I started him back at the beginner level because I wasn't sure what he was capable of any more. He missed four of the ten lessons because of seizures and didn't even get a yellow badge. He was very disappointed, especially as Tara passed her orange and she was two years younger.

I enrolled him in a social skills program at the university. I knew his impulsiveness was not deliberate, but I hoped it might improve his behaviour. It certainly wouldn't hurt him, and maybe the repetition would pay off. Not surprisingly, it didn't. He had already been taught appropriate behaviour at home. He just wasn't able to remember it or act on it. He did enjoy the sessions, though.

The start of the new school year saw Jesse entering grade four. It also heralded one of the worst periods of seizures to date.

It began with a noise in the bedroom. Chris ran, I followed. Jesse was on the floor, completely still, not convulsing. He gave no sign of awareness as Chris picked him up and put him on the bed. We called his name repeatedly, but his eyes remained shut. I pried one eyelid open, then the other. His eyes were still rolled back. He passed from seizure into sleep as we stood beside him, talking worriedly and calling his name. When he finally woke up, he had a terrible headache and a stomach-ache. It was one of the few times he complained of the pain.

The next day after supper, I sent him to take the garbage out. Five minutes later, I asked Chris to check on him. I watched from the kitchen window. Soon they both appeared around the side of the garage, Chris steadying Jesse as he swayed and staggered. His clothes were stained with dirt and grass. There was dirt in his mouth, even in his teeth. His lip was bleeding. I led him to the bathroom, washed his face and mouth, and took off his soiled clothes.

"I'm sorry, Honey. Are you okay?"

"Yeah," he said. "Can I go to bed?"

Labour Day, three days later, began innocuously enough. In the morning he asked if he could go to the store "to buy something." That always meant potato chips, and maybe some candy with the change if he were lucky enough to chisel a dollar out of me. Lately I'd been giving in to his requests for chips, on the grounds that he might actually eat them. He didn't often ask for anything to eat. I knew I would give in this morning, but it was my duty at least to put him off for a while—it's immoral to let your children eat junk food before lunch!

A little later, he asked again, and this time I gave in. "But wait till Tara gets home, and you can go to the store with her."

"I can go by myself."

The store was less than three blocks away.

*He must learn to be independent,* I told myself sternly. *You can't let him see how scared you are.*

*But what if he has a seizure?* I asked myself, equally sternly. *You don't want him to be alone.*

But he wouldn't be alone. Vanscoy is a small town. Everyone knows everyone else, and everyone knew Jesse had seizures.

"Okay," I said. "But watch for cars."

"I know, Mom, you always tell me."

I watched from the kitchen window until he was out of sight. Then I just prayed he'd be all right.

Jesse always took a long time at the store. He could never make up his mind what to buy. Dill pickle chips were a sure thing, but what to get with the change?

He was gone about fifteen minutes before I allowed myself to worry. I phoned the store. They told me he had left five minutes ago. *So he should be home by now.* I checked out the window. I couldn't see him.

"I'll go," said Chris.

I waited anxiously. Jesse had had two *grande mals* in the past four days. I was sure he wouldn't have another one so soon. But I really couldn't be sure of anything.

This time he wasn't walking. Chris was carrying him, like a rag doll. His face was scratched, his clothes dirty. He was almost asleep, his left arm hanging limp.

"He was lying in the dirt," Chris said. "His candy was spread out all across the road."

He fell asleep as soon as I had cleaned him up, and didn't wake up until 1:00. Then he had a strong absence seizure, which left him groggy for a few minutes. An hour later he and Tara walked over to a friend's house to play. Soon afterwards, Bev Turgeon appeared from between two houses across the street. She was carrying a child covered in mud. I knew it was Jesse.

"He's okay," she reassured me. "He had a seizure and fell in the mud. Tara couldn't get him out. She came to me for help."

"I'm so sorry," I said as I took him in my arms. "You're covered in mud."

She waved a hand dismissively. "I'm glad I was there to help."

I carried Jesse into the house. Tara followed, extremely upset.

"I couldn't get him out, Mom."

"It's okay Tara. He's fine." I began to strip off his muddy clothes.

"I didn't know what to do and it was right behind Mrs. Turgeon's house so I went to get her."

"You did the right thing, Tara. That's exactly what you're supposed to do—go and get help."

She still looked distressed.

"Were you worried, Tara?"

She nodded silently and began to cry. I took her in my arms. "It's all right, Tara," I said, reassuring her. "Jesse's fine, everything's fine. It's not your fault. You did the right thing." But I wondered if she was always worried when she was alone with Jesse. I wondered how all this was affecting her—obviously, it was more than I realized.

Jesse was fine for about an hour. Then Tara called from downstairs, telling me that Jesse was having another seizure. It was only an absence, but he had a stronger one half an hour later, and that one knocked him out. I let him sleep for forty minutes, then woke him up to give him his medication. It was almost 5:00. No sooner had he swallowed the pill than he went into another absence. This time he slept for the rest of the night.

Over the next few days, Jesse's seizures became even more frequent. One morning he had two before school, then five more at school. At 3:00 o'clock they called me to come and get him. He had seizures at 3:20, 3:40, 4:00, and 4:45. He slept till 5:55, had another seizure at 6:00, then three more at 6:15, 7:00, and 7:15. He slept until midnight, when he had another.

I called the hospital. The doctor on duty was familiar with Jesse's case. He asked about his last blood levels, and said to increase the Depakene.

Jesse slept in my bed and continued to seize. Several times an hour I was awakened by a small voice: "Mom." All I could do was hold his hands and tell him it would be over soon.

I managed to get Tara off to school in the morning. Jesse woke up at 9:00 and had seven seizures in the next hour and a half. I gave him two Ativans. He had three more seizures before he fell asleep at 11:00. He slept until 2:30. When he woke up he was drugged and slurring his words. He couldn't walk on his own. Finally the seizures began to slow down. He only had ten more that day.

Over the weekend he couldn't eat anything. His weight was falling drastically. I pushed the fluids as much as he would tolerate to keep him from becoming dehydrated. On Monday I managed to get him to eat a bit of Jello. The seizures had begun to slow down, but he'd still had twenty-five by 4:00 o'clock. He was very weak, and looked ghastly.

I knew Dr. Lowry was away until the 25th, but I called his office anyway. There had to be somebody who could stop this. Doris took the information and promised to get back to me. Dr. Bruce called back, saying he would be able to see us in his office at 11:00 the following morning.

Dr. Bruce's manner, as usual, was calm. I didn't want calm. I wanted shock and distress. I wanted someone to be as upset by what Jesse was going through as I was. I knew it was an unrealistic desire, but that didn't stop me from feeling it. Of course, there wasn't anything Dr. Bruce could do. He noted Jesse's pale complexion and his weakness. He checked his blood level.

Dr. Lowry had expressed an interest in seeing the tape of Beth Usher and Brandi Binder. He had never seen a Rasmussen's patient after a hemispherectomy. He'd never seen a Rasmussen's patient at all, in fact, until he met Jesse. I also had papers on Rasmussen's, Chronic Encephalitis, and hemispherectomies, including a chapter of a book Dr. Andermann was writing; he'd given it to me in Montreal the previous summer. All these I now left with Doris, on condition that I get them back. I felt as though I had travelled to the ends of the earth for some of this information.

Before I took Jesse home, we went for lunch. I ordered him a plate of french fries. He was feeling better than he had in a week. If he would eat anything, I thought, fries would be it; they ranked close behind Cheese Whiz toast and dill pickle chips. And it worked. He ate some fries and it seemed to give him strength. By supper time he was able to eat a bit more. He only had five seizures that day.

September continued to be a bad month. Jesse had only two seizure-free days. During the other twenty-eight, he had five *grande mals* in addition to the smaller seizures which numbered anywhere from five to twenty-six a day. On the days he was able to go to school, the staff kept track of his seizures, and let him sleep in the nurse's station afterwards. Some days I was called to pick him up early because he just couldn't manage. Other days I simply kept him home.

He suffered almost constant stomach pain. On the week-end of the 21st he seized every half-hour. Most of them were intense, knocking the starch out of him. Again he slept with me while Chris slept in Jesse's bed. Jesse woke me up every time he felt a seizure coming; we were awake every thirty minutes.

Saturday night, after twenty-six seizures, I gave him an Ativan to try to calm the storm. He slept quite well and I was awakened only once. But on Sunday they continued—fifteen of them. His stomach ached constantly. I kept him home Monday and Tuesday. At school on Wednesday, he had only one absence, but then he was struck down with a *grande mal*.

On Thursday I was booked for day surgery to have an orthoscopy performed on my knee. Arthritis had worn the joint down and it was becoming increasingly painful. It couldn't have come at a worse time. Like everything else, I had been putting it off until Jesse was better. The chances of Jesse ever getting better seemed more remote every time I thought about it. The anti-depressants kept me from going over the edge. Most of the time I was able to carry on, but some days I was just walking through a haze.

The operation went well, but I was on crutches until I could put my full weight on the leg. I sent Jesse to school on Friday, then had to pick him up as he'd hit his head on a wall and again on the floor when he fell while having a seizure. We must have been quite a sight, Jesse and I, as we hobbled out to the car.

*Jo Nanson's Report, October 4th, 1990*

Jesse was cooperative during the assessment, but clearly unwell. He complained of abdominal pain and had one absence seizure lasting sixty seconds during the assessment. He was irritable and needed constant support from his mother to continue the testing. His overall demeanor was very different from the happy, outgoing, overactive child that I saw last year, both here and at his school.

Mrs. Armstrong seemed calmer today. [She mistook exhaustion for calm.] She reported that she is on antidepressants and this seems to help. We had a long conversation after the assessment. I was concerned that she is still hoping that Jesse will be "normal" if he has a hemispherectomy. She cannot seem to accept that Jesse will be left with a dense left hemiplegia and a significant impairment of the intellectual functions served by the right hemisphere.

I will complete psychological testing when Jesse's condition permits.

When I received a copy of this report I was furious. No mother on earth had researched this disease and its possible treatments more thoroughly than I had. I knew as much as anyone—and a great deal more than most—what to expect with a hemispherectomy. I knew what losses would occur, and I certainly was not being unrealistic. I knew Jesse wouldn't be "normal" after the hemispherectomy. I certainly didn't expect a miraculous resurrection of the delightful little boy he had once been. But I knew he would be better than he was.

But what infuriated me most was the fact that I had told no one but her and Chris that I was taking antidepressants. I was not proud of the fact that I needed pills to cope. I certainly didn't want it advertised, especially not to the doctors I had worked so hard to convince that I was informed, knowledgeable, and competent. They had to believe I was voicing my concerns and ruling my decisions with a rational mind.

I felt Jo had betrayed my trust.

I called her a few days later and told her how disappointed and upset I was that she had mentioned me on her assessment. She apologized and explained that the paper would only be going to Dr. Lowry, Dr. Freeman, and me. I didn't know how to tell her that was the whole point, so I let it go.

*Diary entry, October 9th, 1990*

Jesse is sleeping now. He's had a lot of stomach-aches and he's quite dopey. I am assuming it is from the Ativan. I'm very worried. Is the disease confined to the right or not? Are the seizures all originating from the right or not? I'm following most of the doctor's orders, but I have a terrible fear they are steering me off course. I'm really scared now. It's not just a seizure here and there any more. Now the bad hours outweigh the good ones. I feel that it has finally won. The disease has taken hold and I don't know what it will dictate next.

The following day I sent Jesse to school. They called after lunch to say that he was vomiting. Possibly the flu, they said. He had no seizures, but continued to vomit throughout the day. He was weak and dizzy and slept most of the day, waking up only to vomit again.

The next day he began to eat, but I kept him home anyway. The seizures returned—fourteen in all. Friday he wanted to go to school. He had several seizures there and was bothered by stomach-aches for most of the day. On the week-end it was worse. Monday morning I called Dr. Lowry. He said to bring Jesse in for another blood test, but once he took a look at him, he said, "I'll admit him."

Jesse was given five milligrams of Clobezam, a relatively new drug. Dr. Lowry thought it looked promising. At this point, anything was worth a try. Jesse seized every three or four minutes for the rest of the day. The Clobezam made him extremely tired, and he fell asleep in spite of the seizures.

Dr. Lowry dropped in on his rounds early Tuesday morning with four residents.

"Hello, Dr. Lowry," I said, getting up.

"Hello, Nicky. How is Jesse today?"

He had never called me "Nicky" before. It felt unusual, but it felt good, too. Apparently, Jo's evaluation had not had the effect I had feared.

Dr. Lowry turned to the residents. "This is Mrs. Armstrong and Jesse. Jesse was diagnosed with Rasmussen's Encephalitis in Montreal two years ago. Mom here knows an awful lot about this syndrome."

When one doctor treats you with respect, and acknowledges that you *do* have something to contribute, the others follow suit. It was gratifying to know that we were all on the same side, at last.

Jesse stayed in the hospital two more days. On Wednesday the Clobezam seemed to be taking hold. The seizures slowed down, but the medication left him tired and dizzy, much like Ativan had. Thursday morning Dr. Lowry came in and pulled up a chair.

"How is Jesse today?"

"He hasn't had any seizures yet, but he's unsteady when he walks. I have to be beside him constantly."

"We'll decrease the Clobezam to five milligrams twice a day. It will take time for him to adjust. Hopefully, the tiredness will decrease in a few days."

I hoped so, too.

We were discharged later that afternoon. Jesse was still unsteady. I had agreed to give the medication a few days to see if Jesse could adapt to it. It was 5:00 when we arrived home. I helped Jesse to the couch, where he fell asleep immediately. I woke him up at 8:00 to give him his medicine, then put him to bed for the night. At midnight I heard strangled noises coming from his room.

I ran to him. I always ran, never walked. You never get used to the sound of your child in pain.

He was vomiting. His pillow was stained with orange phlegm. He was still sleeping. "Jesse, wake up!" I brought him a bowl and he brought up more. This was scary. *What if he vomits again and begins to choke because he's too drugged to wake up?* I washed him carefully, then carried him back to my bed. This time Chris took the couch.

Ten minutes later I woke up again. Jesse was beside me, his chest and neck heaving. He was vomiting again, and he was still sound asleep.

"Jesse, wake up!" I shook him; he didn't move. "Jesse!"

He looked at me, eyes half closed. "What?" he asked, in a dazed voice.

"You're throwing up in your sleep. I'm taking you to the hospital."

"No, Mom. I'm too tired."

Angry now, I stormed into the living room. "Chris!" I shouted. He sat up with a jerk. "I'm taking Jesse back to the hospital. He's gagging and throwing up while he's still asleep."

I wrapped a blanket around Jesse and put a pillow in the back seat. Chris carried him out to the car, then went back into the house to stay with Tara. I positioned the rear-view mirror so I could see Jesse in the back seat, and I kept talking to him so he wouldn't fall asleep and choke on the way to the hospital.

I burst through the emergency doors, Jesse in my arms. They put him on a gurney in a curtained room while I filled out the appropriate forms. The doctor on duty was already there when I got to Jesse's cubicle.

"Can you tell me what happened, Mrs. Armstrong?" she asked.

"Jesse was just discharged this afternoon. He was sleeping and began to vomit. I brought him to bed with me, and I woke up to him vomiting again. He wasn't even awake. If I hadn't heard him, he could very well have choked. I want you to admit him. Something has got to be done about this medication."

"He's awake now," she said, "and I've checked him. He was sleeping when I came in, but he was easy to rouse. I asked him some questions, and he answered appropriately. You'd better take him home and let him sleep."

"I want you to admit him to the observation unit and keep an eye on him all night. He's so drugged he can't even wake up while he's vomiting. Something has to be done."

"I'm not going to admit him. There's nothing we can do."

"I'm not going home until you do," I said, simply. "You can call Dr. Lowry or whoever you have to. But I will *not* take him home!"

She was angry now. She got up and left the cubicle. When she returned a few moments later, she mumbled, "Dr. Bruce said to observe him overnight. I don't think it's necessary."

I couldn't have cared less what she thought was necessary. I wasn't there at 3:00 in the morning because I had nothing better to do.

Someone came to take Jesse up to the ward. I walked with them, then waited until he was settled. It was 4:00 AM by the time I got back home. At 8:30 the phone rang. Chris answered it.

"It was the hospital," he told me. "Jesse is kicking and fighting and threatening to leave."

"He weighs forty-eight pounds!" I said. "He's too drugged to walk. If he's that feisty all of a sudden, I wish they'd let me in on their secret. Did he throw up in the night?"

"They said he was fine through the night."

"Which nurse did you talk to?"

He told me her name. Then I understood. She was a chronic complainer. She had even complained to me once about other children on the ward. She was a snide and sarcastic woman, and I could not imagine what had led her into a healing profession.

"Chris, could you go to the hospital? I'll get Tara off to school, then I'm going back to bed. I'll be a write-off if I don't get some sleep."

Chris hates hospitals, but he readily agreed.

I slept until 11:00, then went to the hospital. Chris left for work, and I stayed with Jesse. He was still dopey. He stayed in bed most of the time, falling in and out of sleep as his stomach ached. There was no mention in the progress notes about him "kicking and fighting and threatening to leave."

No mention of the nurse having to phone us to control him. All she had written was, "No seizures today. Up ad lib in AM—walks steadily. Very drowsy after 1000 hrs. Father states he is much drowsier & slower than is normal for Jesse. Family visiting. Family spoke to Dr. Lowry and questions were answered."

Dr. Lowry came by at 4:00 PM. He said to reduce the Clobezam to 2.5 milligrams twice a day, continue on Dilantin at 75 milligrams twice a day, and Depakene three times a day: 1000 milligrams, 750 milligrams, and 1000 milligrams.

We talked for a while. I told him about what had happened the night before, and that I was extremely angry with the doctor in emergency. He told me not to worry about it; I had done the right thing. Then I said, "It must have been frustrating for you at first. I know it was for me. Sometimes I felt we were on different sides. It took me a long time to trust you."

"I know it was hard for you," he said. "I was frustrated, too. Many times I thought about Jesse in the evenings, and on week-ends. I wanted to help him."

I thought about that for a few moments, then I said, "It seems that nothing we do makes him any better. He goes through a bad spell with seizures, we do a blood level test. We raise the medication, he gets toxic, he can't eat, he loses weight. We lower the medicine, we change the medicine, the seizures continue. Meanwhile, he's losing ground. He's declining intellectually. And what's happening on the good side of his brain? Is he having seizures from there? What are we accomplishing?"

"It's very frustrating, I agree," he said.

"I spoke to Diana Pillas at Johns Hopkins again in September," I told him. "She said that if things were getting worse, we should look at hemispherectomy. The bottom line, Dr. Lowry, is that I'm scared of the operation, but I'm even more afraid of the damage I'm causing by putting it off. We have to look into it, at least."

"I understand your fears," he replied, "but I believe there's still good function in that hemisphere."

"I can see that there is no hemiparesis," I said, "and his visual fields are both still intact. What I'm saying is, the longer he seizes, the more he'll deteriorate, intellectually and physically. We could let it go until he develops a hemiparesis and loss of visual field on his own. Then, if we do the hemispherectomy, we won't be creating any physical deficit. It will already be there. But how much permanent damage will have been done to the other side? The longer we wait, the greater the chance of him developing a focus for seizures in the good hemisphere. Either way, the infected hemisphere will have to be removed. We have to consider the possibility while there's still something to save."

Dr. Lowry took his time about answering. "I understand what you're saying. But you need to know there will be many more deficits created by the surgery. When a hemispherectomy is done, there is no turning back."

"I know it's a trade-off," I said. "Nothing is free. Right now, seizure control can only be achieved at the expense of large doses of anticonvulsants which have severe side-effects. If we want Jesse to be clear-headed and energetic, we have to lower the doses. Then he suffers more frequent seizures. If we want to stop the deterioration and give him back at least some of his life, then he has to be willing to give up his left arm and left visual field and manage with a weak left leg. That's the trade-off. But what good is a visual field when you're seeing double? And what good is a left arm when you can't use it because you're always either seizing or recovering from a seizure? We're only buying him more time to be sick."

Dr. Lowry listened patiently, but I didn't know if I was getting my point across. Suddenly, he asked, "Would you like me to ask a neurosurgeon here to look at Jesse?"

"Yes," I said, surprised. "I would really appreciate the input."

"Dr. Griebel does most of the pædiatric cases here. I'm not sure when he'll be able to see you. I can't say for sure if he *will* see you, knowing you won't be having the surgery here."

"We only have one chance at this," I said, though I didn't really feel I should have to justify myself. After all, it was my child's life that was at stake. "I want to go where they've done Rasmussen's kids before and have experience with hemispherectomies."

"I'll request a consultation. If he's willing, his office will contact you."

# 16 / In Limbo

Eleven days after Jesse had been discharged from hospital, he was still extremely tired. His teacher's aid came to the house for an hour or two every day to work with him before he fell asleep. He was able to tolerate some food, but he was still very doped. On October 30th I called Dr. Lowry's office and spoke to Doris. "Jesse's still very lethargic," I told her. "His body doesn't seem to be adjusting to the Clobezam. I'm going to cut out the morning dose so he can function during the day."

"How have the seizures been?"

"He hasn't had any since we were in the hospital, but he can't function like this."

"All right, Nicky. I'll check with Dr. Lowry."

When I didn't hear back, I cut out the morning dose the following day. On Halloween, for the first time in weeks, he didn't sleep during the day. I took him to school in the afternoon for the class Halloween party. He had only one small seizure.

That evening he wanted to go trick-or-treating. He made it three blocks before his body gave up on him. I took him home and he slept while Tara and I continued. I gave her Jesse's bag and told her to ask at each door if they would give something for Jesse since he was sick. "People won't mind," I reassured her. "Everybody knows Jesse, and they'll probably ask you where he is."

She rolled her eyes. "It's so *embarrassing*."

Jesse was awake when we returned home, and very grateful to his eight-year-old sister. He gave her a big hug, then rooted through the bag to find his favourite, potato chips. He managed to eat a few, but then his stomach got upset. He was surprised and disappointed that he didn't have the urge to pig out. His Halloween candy lasted a very long time.

November was a write-off. Some days Jesse went to school, but I usually brought him home early. His seizures were less frequent, but he was tired and unsteady all the time. He couldn't remember anything. When someone asked him a question, he seemed to turn it over in his mind, trying to get its meaning. He kept his words to a minimum. He moved slowly, and I often had to help him get dressed. His eyes were vacant. Some days he couldn't walk a straight line. Some days he saw double. He ate enough to maintain his weight, but no more. One day he fell down the back stairs—not from a seizure, but because he'd tripped over his own feet. He was usually in bed for the night by 6:00.

Again I called Dr. Lowry. I told him the situation was not getting any better. "We have seizure control, but he can't think or walk."

"Give it more time," he said, so I did.

Jesse was re-booked with Jo Nanson for November 13th. She began testing him at 9:00 AM. She was surprised at how lethargic he was. She stopped at 11:00, saying we would have to reschedule for another day, as he was too tired to go on.

*Jo Nanson's report*

I saw Jesse on three occasions this fall, October 4th, November 13th, and November 23rd. On November 13th, Jesse appeared heavily sedated and eventually fell asleep during testing.

I had not seen Jesse for a year and was struck by the change in his appearance. He had lost a substantial amount of weight and was pale, with cold extremities. On all three visits, he complained of abdominal pain and nausea. Jesse was hyperactive a year ago and needed constant supervision. On the three visits this year, he was sluggish and very slow to respond. . . .

We went from the Alvin Buckwold Centre to the hospital. "The last blood levels have come back," Dr. Lowry said. "The Dilantin was high. I think we should reduce it."

"He doesn't seem to be tolerating the Clobezam any better than when he first went on it a month ago," I said. "Do you think the dosage is too high?"

"He's on a very small dose," Dr. Lowry said. "Unfortunately, there's no blood test to measure the level. Why don't you reduce the Dilantin now and come back in two weeks for another blood test? If things don't get any better, we'll have to try something else."

A few days later we received a call from Dr. Griebel's office and an appointment date, December 6th.

*Letter from Dr. Lowry to Dr. Griebel, October 31st, 1990*

Jesse has very few motor signs and I think that is why the people in Montreal are reluctant to embark on a hemispherectomy. The people in Baltimore seem more keen as they believe early hemispherectomy is indicated in Rasmussen's Encephalitis. Mother knows that you have some interest and experience in epilepsy surgery and she would value your opinion. I doubt if she seriously plans to have the hemispherectomy done in Saskatoon, but I am just not really sure what is on her mind. She is a very nice lady and knows an awful lot about Rasmussen's Encephalitis. However, she is becoming very depressed and distressed over her son's progressive deterioration. . . .

*Letter to Dr. Freeman from Jo Nanson, November 25th, 1990*

Jesse is showing a global decline in functioning, likely dating back to the onset of his seizure disorder. The results are suggestive of a global encephalopathy, but the most recent testing shows the clearest neuro-psychological evidence of right hemisphere dysfunction. He presently shows defects in attention, verbal and visual memory, strength, fine motor coordination, and constructional abilities.

By the beginning of December Jesse was able to stay awake until seven o'clock. He remained seizure free. He began to eat again, and his stomach seemed fine. It was the best I had seen him in years.

*Diary entry, December 6th, 1990*

Our appointment with Dr. Griebel went well. Jesse was very good. He sat on the examining table and patiently waited for us to speak with the doctor. We talked with him for over an hour. He seemed interested in helping us.

He advised us to come back in a month. Every Tuesday the neurologists and neurosurgeons get together to discuss one interesting case. Dr. Griebel would like us to bring Jesse and together they can come up with some suggestions or opinions. He said he would ask Jo Nanson to be there.

Jesse has been doing extremely well for the past week. He is alert, not tired, having few seizures, and no stomach-aches. His appetite is good and he's eating well. We'll enjoy him now, it won't last forever.

December was a good month. The seizures were at a minimum, nausea was infrequent, and instead of lethargy there was the beginning of a new hyper-activity.

Soon Christmas was upon us. I bought chocolates for Dr. Lowry and his staff, wrapped them carefully, and decorated the box. I enclosed a note, choosing my words carefully. I wanted them to know how much our family appreciated them. Chris's brother, Shawn, spent Christmas with us, and Jesse continued to do well. The seizures were returning, but they weren't as intense as they had been. He was feeling better than he had in a long time. I took the opportunity to speak to him about the surgery.

"Remember how we talked about your seizures?" I asked.

He nodded.

"Do you remember the words 'Rasmussen's Encephalitis'?"

"Yeah, but they don't know why I got it, right?"

"That's right. What happens is that it causes seizures in one side of the brain. The other side is still healthy. The right side of the brain controls the left side of the body, and the left controls the right. So, what side of the brain are your seizures in?"

"Well . . . this arm goes limp, so . . . it would be the right. Right?"

"Right! Now, what the doctors sometimes do to take away the seizures is take out the part of the brain that has the seizures in it. But when they do that, they have to take out the part that controls your left arm and leg. So after that operation your arm stays paralysed and your leg stays weak."

He appeared to understand what I was telling him.

"After this operation," I continued, "most of the kids don't have any more seizures. Some have a few. Do you think it's worth it to get rid of the seizures?"

He thought about it. I didn't tell him that his arm would eventually weaken anyway, even if he didn't have the surgery, or how his seizures were interfering with the functioning of the good side of his brain.

"No," he said simply. "I'd rather have two arms."

That was that, for now.

*Report from pædiatric endocrinologist, Dr. Best, to Dr. Lowry, January 3rd, 1991*

Mother says that Jesse has worn the same clothes for the past three years, and that his shoe size has not increased in a long time. The past year has been a difficult one for Jesse, with seizures more frequent, and associated anorexia and vomiting and consequent weight loss. Mother believes that his abdominal pain comes only as a seizure manifestation and I am inclined to believe she is correct about this.

Jesse does have several other symptoms that are difficult to know how much significance should be attached to them, such as perpetually cold hands and feet and blotchiness of his skin, which seems to occur predominantly during seizure activity. Since beginning Clobezam in mid-October, his seizures have improved, as has his activity level and appetite.

In summary, then, I believe that Jesse's relatively slow growth has a nutritional basis, which is in turn secondary to his Rasmussen's Encephalitis with its frequent seizures and impact on his appetite and gastrointestinal function. I do not believe that his past steroid therapy has had a significant deleterious effect on his growth.

On January 13th Dr. Lowry called. He thanked me for the chocolates and card and told me Dr. Griebel had set up a neurology conference on January 22nd. I told him that Jesse was better than he'd been in a long time. Dr. Lowry seemed pleasantly surprised.

"I wonder if we should go ahead with the conference," I said. "Jesse is definitely still sick, but he's doing so much better than he was a couple of months ago."

"I think we should go ahead, anyway," Dr. Lowry said, and went on to explain the procedure: "The conference will be dealt with in two parts. In the first forty-five minutes, I'll be introducing Rasmussen's Encephalitis in general, then discussing Jesse's case in particular. Jo Nanson will be there to review the neuro-psychological aspects of the disease. After that, we'll bring Jesse in."

I desperately wanted to sit in on the first part, but I didn't ask him. I didn't like to push my luck.

"By the way," he said, "would you like to sit in on the first part?"

Jo Nanson had spoken with Diana Pillas at Johns Hopkins. She told me Dr. Freeman had consulted with his team and concluded that we should consider hemispherectomy now. They all felt Jesse would benefit from it. Dr. Freeman also said that it would be best to have the surgery done locally. A competent neurosurgeon with a good OR staff was the first consideration. The next was family support, which he believed was instrumental in the recovery of the patient. A third consideration was that Jesse would need frequent physical therapy afterwards. Jo suggested I call Diana to discuss these concerns further. When I did, Diana merely confirmed to me what she had said to Jo. It was great that Jesse was doing so much better, she said, but it wouldn't last.

The neurology conference was on January 22nd. I didn't learn anything new, but I was grateful to have been included. I called Dr. Griebel later that day.

"Dr. Lowry and I have come to the conclusion," he said, "that if Jesse runs into another bad bout with seizures, we should seriously consider the operation. Because he's doing so well at the moment, though, we should put it off for the time being."

"That's what I think," I told him.

"I appreciate the fact that you've kept such a complete and concise diary of Jesse's deterioration," he went on. "It was extremely helpful in my assessment and in making my recommendations."

That was good to hear, too.

In February and March the shake-out seizures and arm jerks increased, but they were nowhere near the level they had been in the fall. Jesse's impulsiveness was a problem, however, and he continued to regress socially.

At the end of March, Chris and I went to the school one afternoon for the annual Science Fair. Jesse's teacher, Mrs. Johnson, approached us. She looked very serious. "Could I speak with you for a few minutes?"

She ushered us into the grade four classroom and shut the door.

"There was an incident this morning," she said. "Jesse was outside before class, and he attacked Kim for no reason."

"What?"

"He grabbed her from behind and pulled her down. He wouldn't let go of her hat."

"Are you sure?" I asked in disbelief. "I know Jesse's impulsive, but he's not mean." Then I asked, "Is Kim all right? Is she hurt?"

Eyes downcast, Mrs. Johnson said, "She was quite shaken, but I spoke to her and she's all right now. I had Jesse apologize to her."

"Are you *sure*?" I asked again. The idea of Jesse attacking anyone was preposterous, I thought. But then, I didn't really know him any more. I'd heard of people becoming violent after suffering brain damage.

"Kim's mother was driving away when it happened. She was honking the horn to get someone's attention."

My heart sank. Impulsiveness and disinhibited behaviour were one thing, but aggression was a different matter. I had tried so hard to keep the last fragments of the Jesse I knew. But he was gone now.

"I'll speak to Jo Nanson," I said. I didn't know what else to say. I was on the verge of tears.

As soon as I got home, I started making phone calls. I called Jo first. I told her about the incident, and booked an appointment. Then I called the neuro-psychologist I had spoken to in Montreal, but he wasn't available.

I cried as I waited for Jesse to come home from school. I would ask him why he did it. I would demand to know. I would insist that it never happen again.

But it wouldn't matter. I could demand; I could insist. The disease demanded with a stronger voice. Every time I thought things couldn't get any worse, they got worse. *That's it,* I thought. *This disease has overpowered every aspect of my boy. I have no control. It's all chance and fate.*

When Jesse finally came home, he behaved as if nothing happened. As soon as he was in the door I started in on him.

"What happened in school today?" I demanded.

"Nothing."

His nonchalance infuriated me. "Something happened with Kim!" I shouted. "Tell me what happened!"

He was scared now. "I just pulled her hat off at recess."

"Mrs. Johnson said you attacked her and her Mom had to beep her horn for someone to help! What the hell were you doing?"

He was scared and confused—scared of me yelling at him, but what was he confused about? Tara stood, scared and silent. She had witnessed scenes like this before.

"I was just playing, Mom."

"Just playing? Attacking someone and pulling them down is *just playing*? How many times have I told you to keep your hands to yourself! You're *not* to touch people! What am I going to do with you?"

"I'm sorry," he said. "I'm sorry."

I sent him to his room, then went down to the office in the basement and closed the door. I knew I had to phone Kim's mother. I thought of sending Jesse over to apologize in person, but I didn't know how upset she would be.

I had always encouraged kids to come over. I often gave Jesse and his companions treats when they were playing. I tried to make them like it here, so they would come back. Jesse wasn't interested in anything but playing. He wanted friends, but he didn't know how to keep them. Now this. How could I control this?

The simple answer was, I couldn't.

I spent some time rehearsing what I would say to Kim's mother, then I dialled the number.

"It's Nicky Armstrong," I said. "Is Kim okay?"

"Well . . . yes." She sounded surprised. "I think so."

I took a deep breath. "The teacher told us that Jesse had hurt her." I couldn't use the word *attacked.* "I'm really sorry. Did you see what happened?"

"Sure. I'd just dropped Kim off at school and there were a bunch of kids outside. I started driving away when I saw Jesse pulling on Kim and grabbing at her hat."

"Mrs. Johnson said you were honking your horn to get help."

"Well, not really. He kept pulling on her hat, so I just beeped the horn as I drove off so he'd see me and stop."

"You didn't stop the car?"

"No, he was just bugging her. He wasn't hurting her."

"That's not the impression I got from Mrs. Johnson. She said that Jesse attacked Kim and you were honking the horn to get someone's attention to help."

"He was just trying to pull her hat off. After I honked the horn, he stopped. I drove away."

"I'm sorry if he hurt her," I said, and I started crying again.

"Don't worry about it. He didn't."

I put down the receiver. I was crying in anger this time—at Mrs. Johnson for blowing the episode out of proportion. Now I had to apologize to Jesse. I went back upstairs.

"Jesse," I said, "I'm sorry for yelling at you. Mrs. Johnson made it sound worse than it was. But, still, you can't be grabbing people. You have to keep your hands to yourself."

"I'm sorry, Mom," he said.

"I'm sorry, too."

He never thought twice about forgiving me for distrusting him, or for yelling at him. He was annoying and impulsive, and he teased too much. Still, I had a few things to learn from him. So did other people, I thought.

I couldn't let go of the anger. When the teacher's aid called me a few days later to report on Jesse's seizures, I was still fuming. I told her how angry I was with Mrs. Johnson. I couldn't understand how she could have viewed the incident so differently than Kim's mother, who was surely more concerned about Kim's welfare. It was then I learned that no teacher, including Mrs. Johnson, had even witnessed the incident. It was another grade four student who had reported it to Mrs. Johnson. Jesse was asked if he had knocked Kim down and pulled off her hat. He replied truthfully, and was brought to apologize to Kim. Mrs. Johnson then misrepresented the incident as an unprovoked attack.

At my appointment with Jo Nanson, we spoke for two hours. Jo said she would speak to the school and give them some ideas on behaviour modification.

*Note to Dr. Lowry from Jo Nanson, April 30th, 1991*

I visited Vanscoy School today at Mrs. Armstrong's request. Jesse had been disrupting the class and difficult at lunch time and recess. We discussed some behaviour management techniques.

The teachers were surprised to learn that Jesse's brain functioning is not "normal" even when he is not seizing, and that the abdominal pains are likely seizures.

The school has tested him again (I'm not sure why, or how valid the testing is as the school teacher is not qualified to do the tests). The results were described as similar to mine in November—i.e., he is not catching up again but is not regressing.

When I found out about the testing, I called the principal and told him that they were not to do any testing without my permission. Because the psychological tests could not be repeated for at least six months, preferably a year, the school had set us back at least another six months.

*Letter to Cindy and Steven Binder, April 1st, 1991*

I don't know what to do. When I see Jesse feeling well, playing baseball and having only the odd seizure, I think I will never ever let him have the operation, unless he were to die if he didn't. But, when I look at the overall picture and evaluate his life and quality of life, and think of his future, I wonder if I'm not doing his future more harm by denying him a hemispherectomy.

It seems every Rasmussen's patient has ended up with a hemispherectomy at some point. They speak of burn out, but I have not actually heard of any valid case. Are we losing precious time?

Each seizure may be doing permanent damage to the good left hemisphere. A lot of Jesse's neuro-psychological tests come out showing more global damage. If we wait too long could a focus for seizures begin in the left? Not the encephalitis itself, but what if when we do the hemispherectomy, we have let him seize too much and waited so long that we end up with seizures from the left because it has developed a focus. So then he ends up with a hemispherectomy, hemiparesis, loss of left visual field, and still he has seizures and is on anticonvulsants for the rest of his life.

Another very definite worry is that his IQ is steadily dropping each year. Wouldn't it be better to do surgery while he still has a high IQ and lose less? I feel these are points which will never be regained. If we had had surgery when his IQ had dropped to ninety-six instead of now at seventy-six, wouldn't he have been better off to start his healing at that point?

How far do we let it drop before we stop the encephalitis? It may sound like I am in favour of hemispherectomy. It really is that I am almost more afraid of the alternative, which is waiting for paralysis and watching more irreversible deterioration.

I'm scared to death of hemispherectomy, but I'm also scared to death to sit idle.

No one seems to be able to advise us on this. The doctors do not recommend hemispherectomy because they see no left-sided weakness and know how much will be lost. But, on the other hand, they do believe that the younger the patient, the easier it is to transfer function and so on. . . . No one wants to commit themselves. I can see why. There is too much to lose, either way.

I think it is harder to keep a proper perspective when you are dealing with a slowly progressive encephalitis than a faster, more intense one. I feel guilty wishing the disease would either get worse fast or stop altogether. We are all tired of being in limbo, just worrying about Jesse's future but not really being able to start planning it. I feel that I don't understand any of it any more. I don't know if I'm making any sense to you. I would like your opinion. Would you have these same worries, or should we just be thankful that he is not forced to have a hemispherectomy just now and just forget about all the "what ifs"?

I just don't understand how something like this could have happened to our healthy babies. I have read that God only gives "special needs" children to very "special" families, and that He will never give us more than we can handle. I hope I don't disappoint Him. I guess we all get weary of being the chosen ones.

# 17 / "Got My Own Wheels"

Jesse had gained nearly ten pounds over five months, and he was maintaining it. Even with this gain, however, he was still below average for his age. Then, in the first week of May his appetite began to decrease again. A week later he came home from school, his lunch kit unopened. He was weak, and his eyes were rimmed with red. He went to the couch and lay down.

"We have to take Tara to her baseball game in an hour," I told him.

"Can't I stay home?"

"No, Dad won't be home before we leave."

"My stomach hurts."

He looked as if he'd been through the wringer. How could I make him sit through a baseball game when all he wanted was to lie down? I arranged for him to stay at Turgeon's until Chris got home. When Tara and I returned at 8:00, Jesse was in bed. I asked Chris the usual questions.

"When did he fall asleep?"

"About 6:30. He said he felt like throwing up. He wouldn't eat any supper."

"Any seizures?"

"Just a few shake-outs."

"I wonder what's wrong now?"

"Probably just allergies," Chris reassured me. "Wait and see how he is tomorrow."

"Tomorrow" arrived at 1:30 AM. I was used to hearing Jesse moan in the night, but this was different. This was a scream. I jumped out of bed and rushed to his room.

"Ow, my stomach!" he cried. "*My stomach!*"

"Show me exactly where it hurts."

He moved his hand over his belly. "I'm going to throw up."

I rushed to the kitchen for a bowl. No sooner had I returned than he began to heave. But he could only bring up bile and saliva. He had eaten nothing since breakfast.

I was at a loss. His seizures weren't frequent enough to cause such a reaction. He was slow and weak, but he wasn't bumping into walls or falling from toxicity. These pains were far more severe than his usual stomach-ache seizures but, like the seizures, they were intermittent.

I was able to get him in to see Dr. Lowry that afternoon. It was obvious that something was wrong, but Dr. Lowry, too, was unsure of the cause. He did a blood level test and sent Jesse to have an EEG. He walked in the EEG room while Jesse was still being monitored.

"The Epival is very high," he said. "The range is 700 to 900. Jesse's at 1450. It looks like he may have developed pancreatitis. We'll reduce the Epival immediately. The pain should decrease in a day or two."

Jesse was awake on and off throughout the night. Again Chris slept in Jesse's room while Jesse stayed with me. He would sleep for a few minutes, then wake up with cramps, crying with pain until they abated and he fell back asleep. I, too, slept between the cramps. Each time I awoke with a start as he cried out. I couldn't comfort him; the pain was too intense. He brought his knees to his stomach and curled up in the fetal position. He kept one hand on his stomach and reached for me with the other, gripping tightly until the pain went away. Then he fell asleep for another minute or two.

By 2:00 AM I couldn't stand it any longer, and called the hospital. The resident on duty was familiar with Jesse's case. He suggested I give him Tylenol every four hours. I gave him one immediately. It took about twenty minutes to take effect, then he was able to sleep for a blessed hour and a half. After that, it was another two and a half hours of pain until I could give him another dose.

At 8:30 I called Dr. Lowry's office. I knew he was away for the long week-end, but he had introduced me to Dr. Earl the day before. Dr. Earl was a resident, and familiar with Jesse's case. He advised me to give him as much liquid as he could tolerate. "If he isn't feeling better by tomorrow, bring him in. I'll put him on an IV to give him liquids and a pain reliever."

"The Tylenol only works for an hour and a half," I said, "then he's in severe pain until I can give him another. What do I do if he gets worse?"

"We eliminated the Epival yesterday, so the pain should decrease soon. If things get worse, call emergency and speak to the pædiatric resident on duty. I'll check tonight's schedule and inform them that you may be calling."

The pain continued throughout the night. The cramps lessened somewhat in intensity, but their frequency and duration remained the same. Again

I called the hospital. The resident on duty was not surprised about the pain. "Pancreatitis is extremely painful. It takes a while for the pancreas to heal. In the meantime, continue with the Tylenol. I'm more concerned about dehydration. If you think he's not drinking enough, bring him in to be fed intravenously. I'm afraid that's all we can do at this point."

The following day he felt better. The pain had decreased substantially, and he was able to eat a small amount. The stomach-aches were more of the seizure type now than the intense pain that had been doubling him up over for the past few days. I put him in his own bed that night, and went to bed early myself, looking forward to a good night's sleep for the first time in three days.

It was not to be. In the middle of the night he called me, not from his bedroom but from the bathroom. He was standing, obviously in pain, his pyjamas and the floor covered in excrement.

"What happened?"

"I don't know," he said. "I got a stomach-ache."

"Don't worry, honey. We'll get you cleaned up."

I gave him a quick bath, rinsed his clothes and washed the floor, then put him back to bed. He slept for the rest of the night, but he didn't look good when he woke up. The cramps were back. At noon he went into an intense seizure, and fell asleep immediately afterwards. He woke up at 2:30, only to go into another. As I waited for it to subside, he went into convulsions. He slept on and off between the cramps, all day and evening. He had another four *grande mals* before midnight. He was running a fever of 101º F.

Once again I took him to bed with me. I continued to give him Tylenol, but the pain did not subside. At 1:30 AM I awoke to the repetitive gasps and jerking of a *grande mal*. I pulled him onto his side and moved the pillow to give him a good airway. Once the seizure had subsided I replaced his pillow and positioned his limp left arm so it would be comfortable when the feeling returned.

He went into convulsions again at 3:30, then again at 6:00. I let him sleep for a while after the last one, then I got him dressed to go to the hospital. He had another *grande mal* on the way, and was asleep when I arrived. They took him to a curtained cubicle and put him on a gurney with the side rails up.

I filled out the necessary forms and went to him. He was awake, but still had stomach pain. I lowered the left rail and stood over him as a resident took his history. At 8:15 he began to stare. I told the resident that he was going to have a seizure. Another *grande mal*. I turned him on his side and stood by him while the storm continued. When it was over, I wiped his mouth and made him comfortable, then covered him and continued to speak to the doctor.

Soon Dr. Lowry walked in. "He's still got cramps," I told him. "And now he's having *grande mals*—ten since yesterday."

"We have to get these seizures under control," Dr. Lowry said. "I'll have Dr. Bruce look at him again. I have to get his file from my office. Come with me. We'll talk on the way."

I looked at the resident questioningly. "I'll stay right here," he reassured me. I followed Dr. Lowry up to pædiatrics.

"Dr. Bruce and I are not entirely convinced that the diagnosis of pancreatitis is correct," he said. "Jesse's urinary calcium is elevated, and we're wondering if that could be the cause of his pain. We aren't sure of the cause, but we know that his pain is very real."

I carried Jesse's file back to emergency with me. Dr. Lowry stayed in pædiatrics, for he had interrupted his morning rounds to look in on us.

At 10:10 AM, Jesse's eyes once again glazed over. The convulsions began quickly, and they were more severe. I didn't have time to put him on his side. He was well into the seizure when I noticed Terry from EEG walking by. I called to him, and he rushed over and gave me a hand. Then he stood by until the convulsions had stopped.

Forty-five minutes later, Jesse again went into convulsions. A doctor tending another patient nearby looked up, concern in his face. "Do you need help?"

"He'll be okay," I said. "We're just waiting to be admitted."

When the storm had subsided, the doctor called to a nurse who was rushing by. "Put this boy on oxygen"—he pointed—"now, please!"

The nurse abandoned whatever she had been doing and came to Jesse's bedside. She took the oxygen mask from the wall and placed it over his mouth and nose. Jesse, eyes still closed, tried to push it off. "They're just giving you oxygen, Jesse," I told him. He dropped his hand and fell into a deep sleep.

We were on the ward by 11:00, admission papers filled out and history taken yet again. He was kept on oxygen and put on a cardiac monitor. Ten minutes later he went into another convulsive seizure. Dr. Lowry ordered five milligrams of Clobezam to be given immediately.

Jesse had another seizure at 1:00 and another at 1:45. They were intense and long, but neither developed into convulsions.

Another *grande mal* at 3:25. We were still waiting to see Dr. Bruce. The resident hadn't been in yet.

Another at 4:45. I went to the nursing station. "I want to see a doctor. We have to stop these seizures."

"The resident should be up shortly."

"Where's Dr. Lowry?"

"I'm not sure if he's gone for the day. He may still be in pædiatrics," she said. "I'll page the resident."

I walked back to Jesse's room. He was sound asleep. He slept until another *grande mal* woke him at 5:30.

At 5:45 the resident finally walked in. "Dr. Lowry has asked that an intravenous be started. We'll give him a loading dose of Dilantin. Hopefully that'll stop the seizures."

Jesse had one more *grande mal* fifteen minutes later. The cardiac monitor raced. I held onto the arm that was hooked up to the IV to make sure the needle didn't come out.

The next seizure, an hour later, was intense but not convulsive. I stayed until he was asleep for the night.

The next day the cramps weren't nearly as intense. Every time one came he felt an urgency to urinate. His urine had a high calcium count, which meant that the pain he was experiencing was comparable to that experienced with gallstones. To flush out the calcium, I began giving him water or juice every half hour.

The following day Jesse was just finishing his breakfast when I arrived. He looked great. He was discharged at 11:00, the seizures once again under control, the cramps nearly gone. He went to school for the first time in over a week. The crisis was over—this crisis, anyway.

Dilantin was the anticonvulsant used in the hospital because it can be given intravenously. The medication Jesse was given on discharge was Clobezam. Both dosages were raised. He was now on five milligrams of Clobezam three times a day and seventy-five of Dilantin twice a day.

He started having headaches a few days after being released. I took him in for a blood level test and asked Dr. Lowry about putting him back on Epival, since it seemed to control his seizures better than Dilantin. If he maintained a high fluid intake, I thought, it should be safe. Dr. Lowry said it would take two weeks to wean Jesse off Dilantin.

The transition was not easy. His appetite began decreasing again. He continued to have shake-outs and arm jerks; it was not uncommon for him to have fifty to a hundred of these small seizures every day. By July 17th he was off Dilantin and on a maintenance dose of 1000 milligrams a day of Epival. But things weren't getting any better. Every day there were seizures, and more seizures.

I wondered where it was all going. I wondered why it had happened in the first place, and if it would ever stop. I watched the neighbourhood children playing outside while Jesse slept after a seizure, or while he sat watching TV with a bowl and a box of tissues. I tried to remember exactly when it was that I had accepted this life for him. When exactly did all of these unnatural acts become natural to him, and to me?

In bed at night, Chris and I spoke about surgery. Sometimes we both agreed it was the best and only thing to do to save Jesse, to give him a future. He was still regressing, intellectually and emotionally. We were afraid for his future, and our hearts ached for his present: the bumps, the bruises, the stomach-aches, the seizures, the headaches, the nausea. At other times we felt we could never do such a radical thing to our son, no matter how sick he got. Every good day reinforced this conviction; every bad day weakened it.

One Saturday Chris and Jesse came home from Saskatoon with a garage sale purchase. Jesse stepped out of the car with a huge smile on his face. "Mom, look what Dad bought for me!" he exclaimed as Chris took a blue two-wheeled scooter out of the trunk. I gave Chris a disapproving look. We had decided years ago that a bike was too dangerous. Was this any different? But I couldn't tell them to take it back. Not yet. Not in front of Jesse. He was too happy. He pushed the scooter onto the road. "Got my own wheels," he said excitedly. "See, I can ride it. It's got hand brakes, too."

I stood with a smile on my face and my heart in my mouth.

"Okay, Jesse," Chris said, "we'll clean it up and oil it before you ride it. Put it in the garage for now. We'll start working on it in a few minutes."

As soon as Jesse was out of hearing, I said, "Chris, he can't ride that. It's too dangerous."

"He wanted it so badly, Nicky. I thought about the danger, too, but it doesn't go very fast and the footboard's only four inches off the ground. He'll be travelling slower on the scooter than if he was running."

Chris was right. Jesse was at risk wherever he was, on a scooter or on foot. The pleasure he would get from it, the independence he would feel: surely these were worth the risks. He hadn't had wheels since he was five.

In August we went to Calgary for a vacation. Jesse's stomach cramps were returning and his appetite was low, so I made sure that I knew which hospital to go to should we run into difficulties. Jesse had stomach-aches most days, but they were not the strong cramps he had experienced in May. He was having shake-out seizures and a few absences, but when we took him and Tara to Calaway Park, they both loved it.

It wasn't until we started on the long drive home that the cramps returned with the intensity that had crippled him before. From Oyen to

Rosetown, he spent much of the time curled up against the window, holding his stomach and wincing. He slept through the night once we got home, but the cramps woke him again at 6:00 AM. I took him in for an EEG and CT scan that Dr. Lowry had booked before we left. The pain subsided throughout the day, but returned toward evening. I put him in my bed, anticipating another all-nighter. I put a bowl, a box of tissues, and a glass of juice on the night table, and used each in turn through the night. It was critical to keep his fluid intake up.

He spent the next day on the couch, feeling sick, and that night the cramps got much worse. By 3:00 AM I was beside myself with anxiety and concern for my child. I called the hospital. Other than giving Jesse Tylenol, the resident on call said, they could do nothing for him. We'd just have to wait until Dr. Lowry arrived in the morning. I watched the clock between cramps. Dr. Lowry was probably getting out of bed and having his breakfast as I dressed Jesse and drove him to the hospital.

They took more blood and another urine sample. Again there was calcium in his urine. I was to push the fluids more to flush it out. Dr. Bruce gave us a bottle for a twenty-four hour urine sample. I was to bring it back Monday morning. Today was Friday.

Jesse was in agony all through Friday night. I gave him Tylenol every four hours. By Saturday the pain seemed to subside. I put him to bed at 8:30 Saturday night. Shortly afterwards, he came to me in the living room.

"Mom, there's something wrong with my left arm."

There was, indeed. His left shoulder drooped, and his arm hung lifeless.

"Did you have a big seizure?" I asked.

"My arm was jumping in bed and now I can't move it," he said. He wasn't scared. He was merely stating a fact.

The fingers were limp and the arm was cold. I knew he couldn't have had a *grande mal* because he would not have remembered it. There was no point calling the hospital. I knew what they'd say: "Is he in a seizure?" "No." "Then wait till Monday and see Dr. Lowry."

The paralysis lasted about five minutes, then the feeling gradually returned. I sent him back to bed. I didn't know what had happened and I didn't know what to do about it. I was exhausted. I couldn't think any more.

The cramps continued through the night. On Sunday I became the water police. I made him finish a full glass every hour. He only woke up twice that night with cramps.

I took his twenty-four hour urine sample in to the hospital. Dr. Lowry could find nothing wrong with it, other than the high calcium content. He said to continue pushing the fluids, it seemed to be helping. By Monday afternoon the cramps were nearly gone.

Later that day Chris and the kids were working in the yard. Tara was helping with the mowing and Jesse was edging the lawn with the electric snipper. I was in the house, cleaning up after lunch. It felt good to have Jesse off the couch and getting some fresh air. I was grateful that he seemed to be feeling better. I'd had a fairly good sleep myself the night before, only waking twice to Jesse's cramps.

Suddenly through the window I heard, "Jesse!"

It was Tara's voice, and I knew he was down. I ran to the back door. Jesse was stuck between a tree and the fence, his head and arm jerking rhythmically. The electric snipper had landed two feet away.

Two days later he had another *grande mal*. When he had recovered from that, I approached him again about surgery.

"Remember when we talked about the operation that would take away your seizures but leave you with a paralysed arm?" I asked.

"Yes," he said.

"What do you think about that now?"

"They can't take away my seizures and leave my hand?"

I swallowed my anger. It was so unfair! My son was being asked to give up his left arm and part of his leg in exchange for a semi-normal life, a life that every child should be entitled to.

"No, honey. The seizures are in the part of the brain that controls your arm."

He thought about it some more. Then, for the first time, he said, "I want the operation. I want to get rid of all these seizures and stomach-aches. I guess I could still do things with one hand."

I set up a family conference with Dr. Lowry and Dr. Griebel. I asked my sisters Henriette and Jeanne to sit in on it. I needed objective opinions. Maybe they could see something that Chris and I couldn't.

When the time came, everyone took a turn asking questions. Then we discussed Jesse's illness and deterioration, the objective of the surgery, and both the benefits of and the drawbacks to performing it early instead of waiting for the hemiparesis and hemianopsia (visual field defect) to come first. Dr. Lowry concluded that surgery would definitely be of benefit to Jesse now. With seizure control, we could stop the deterioration and allow for better intellectual growth. The disadvantages, of course, would be the premature creation of both the hemiparesis and the hemianopsia.

"First," he continued, "we must determine whether Jesse's seizures are all originating from the right hemisphere, and second, whether speech is served by the unaffected left hemisphere."

Ninety percent of people have speech representation in the left hemisphere. The likelihood is even higher when the individual is right-handed. But Dr. Lowry wanted to perform a Wada test to be absolutely certain. The test consisted of injecting sodium amytol into the artery serving the right hemisphere. The drug would render the hemisphere unconscious. If Jesse was still able to produce speech, we would then be certain that his representation was indeed in the left hemisphere.

To determine the definite origin of the seizures, Dr. Lowry would put Jesse on telemetry for several days until he had recorded a sufficient number of seizures for a thorough investigation of their origin.

I left the office with renewed hope for a better life for Jesse. At the same time, not unnaturally, I was extremely apprehensive. I felt a surge of panic at the thought of removing half my son's brain. Did I have any idea what I was really assenting to?

A short while later, the University Book Store called to say that Dr. Andermann's book, *Chronic Encephalitis and Epilepsy (Rasmussen's Syndrome)*, was finally available. I didn't care what the cost, I was going to have a copy. I met my sister Henriette at the University and bought the book. She then took me to the medical library, where I photocopied the few recent publications on the syndrome.

Jesse was scheduled for telemetry October 2nd. This would tell the tale. It would be the deciding factor as to whether or not we proceeded with a hemispherectomy.

# 18 / Decision

August 28th: the first day of a new school year. Jesse was going into grade five, Tara into grade four. Jesse was anxious to take his new wheels to school. I went over the procedure with Tara, telling her what to do if Jesse had a seizure on the way. Then the two of them headed out, Tara on her bike and Jesse on his scooter. I held my breath until 9:00 o'clock. When the phone didn't ring, I knew they'd made it to school without incident.

At 3:30 I started watching for them. When I could see them down the street, I heaved a sigh of relief and moved away from the window so they wouldn't see me.

They came in full of news and excitement. It was wonderful.

The second day, I had just begun my 3:30 vigil at the window when the phone rang. It was my neighbour, Nancy. "Your little guy just had an accident!" Her voice was distressed, almost panicky. "He's on the road in front of my place!"

"I'll be right there."

I knew by the sound of her voice that I would need the car to bring Jesse home. When I backed out of the driveway I saw a circle of kids on the road ahead. Jesse's scooter lay by the side of the road. I threw the gear shift into park even before the car had stopped, and jumped out. Tara was crying hysterically on the side of the road. I pushed through the circle of kids to reach her. Then I saw Jesse. His head was covered in blood. His chest heaved with soft convulsions, and his breathing was ragged. Nancy was beside him, pale and trembling, not knowing what to do.

Tara was crying uncontrollably. "Honey, it's okay," I said. "I'll take care of him." I knew she needed me, but Jesse's need was more immediate. I turned to a friend nearby. "Would you walk Tara home? She's very upset."

I wasn't sure where Jesse was bleeding. From the amount of blood it looked as if his head had split open. He was still unconscious as I lifted him from the ground. "It's okay, honey-bear," I said in a shaky voice. "You're going to be okay."

"I'll drive," Nancy said, jumping into the driver's seat. "You get in the back with Jesse."

We met Chris running toward us. A child had rung the doorbell and told him, "Jesse had a seizure down the road and split his head open." But Jesse was beginning to moan, and I knew he'd be all right. Chris scooped him from my arms and carried him into the house. I thanked Nancy, and reassured her Jesse would be okay.

Once we had washed off the blood, we could see the cut, a deep gouge above his right eyebrow. His right ear and cheek were scraped. Other than that he seemed all right.

Tara was in her room, still crying, her face buried in her pillows.

"Honey, it's okay," I said. "Jesse's going to be okay."

"Mom, I thought he was going to die!"

I took her in my arms. "I know it looked bad, but he's just got a little cut. I'm going to take him in for a couple of stitches."

"I couldn't catch him," she sobbed.

I held her by her shoulders and looked her in the eye. "Tara, it's not your fault!" She continued to cry. "Listen to me, Tara. It was an accident. You can't catch him when he has these seizures! No one can. They happen too fast!"

"I didn't know what to do."

"You did exactly the right thing. You got someone to call me, and you stayed with him until I came. That's all anyone could have done. He's going to be just fine."

"*But he isn't!*" she screamed. "I can't *stand* it! When is it going to stop?"

I could only hold her while she cried. I knew exactly how she felt.

Jesse ended up with a couple of stitches. I held his hand while the emergency clinic doctor (who turned out to be Dr. Lowry's wife— small world) injected the freezing directly into the wound. Jesse accepted it without complaint. I wondered if this marvellous compliance of his was God's compensation to us for all he had to endure.

Later that afternoon, Nancy and her husband came over to see how Jesse was. They were deeply concerned, and Nancy was still upset by the incident. I had become so used to this way of life that it took me aback when someone like Nancy reminded me how a normal person responds to an abnormal situation.

Normality, now, was living on the edge. The following day, Jesse's note from school reported that he'd had ten seizures between 9:00 and 10:00 AM alone. He continued to have frequent small seizures throughout September, with one *grande mal* on the 3rd, another on the 4th, and a third on the 6th. The paralysis that time stayed longer than usual, and the left side of his face, he said, felt "strange."

Later that same day, a child came to the door and told me that Jesse had had a seizure. He led me to where Jesse was lying. There was a truck on the road, the door open. A man was standing over Jesse. My heart stopped.

I ran as only a mother can run when she sees her child in danger. To my great relief, I saw that he had not been hit by the truck. The driver had kindly stopped to help when he saw Jesse go down.

Safe for one more day.

Wednesday, October 2nd, we began the telemetry tests to determine the definite origin of the seizures. They were the same tests he'd had in Baltimore. We were settled in a private room and a technician came up with the EEG machine. He pasted the now familiar electrodes systematically on Jesse's scalp. He strapped the power box to a belt that could be put around Jesse's waist, leaving his hands free if he felt like moving around.

He had several shake-out seizures, but they were so short I barely had time to press the button to mark the tape. I was told then to mark only the stronger seizures.

Wednesday passed into Thursday, and Thursday ground on. Jesse continued to have small seizures and stomach-aches, but none that lasted any length of time. They brought in a TV to relieve the boredom. I left the room only for a coffee break or a meal. We spent the days playing cards and other games. At one point, I casually asked, "Jesse, guess what?"

"What?" he asked, without looking up.

"Love you!" I laughed. "I finally got you!"

We played this game often, but it was rare to catch him off guard.

"I knew you were going to say that," he said. He tried to keep a straight face, but he couldn't hide the smile. "I'll get you next time," he promised.

Late on Thursday afternoon, Dr. Lowry came by. "Anything today?"

"Nothing but shake-outs," I said.

"Don't worry, they'll come. Often when you put a seizure patient on telemetry the seizures stop altogether or drop dramatically in frequency. If we don't see any significant seizures by tomorrow afternoon when you leave for the week-end, I'll get you to reduce his medication on Sunday before you come back. I'm not worried about being unable to record enough seizures, not with Jesse."

On Friday we continued to play cards, watch television, and read stories. It felt odd to be disappointed that Jesse wasn't having any *grande mals*. Then, just before we were to leave for the week-end, Jesse's right hand suddenly hit the bed table while we were playing cards. His body stiffened, and he fell backwards. I pushed the button immediately, then struggled to keep him on the bed, checking the monitor to make sure as much as possible that he was on camera and I wasn't.

As I watched him convulse, I noticed that his eyes were up and to the right. *That can't be right,* I thought. I checked again. His eyes were definitely to the right. I'd never seen that before. *He always turns to the left and his eyes are always to the left. If they're going to the right,* I reasoned, *it must mean this seizure is originating in the left hemisphere. The good hemisphere.*

When Rita the technician came in later to remove the electrodes, I told her about the seizure and bombarded her with questions. I asked to see Dr. Lowry, but he was still seeing patients in his office. I was near panic, and crying by the time we got home.

"What are we going to do now?" I asked Chris. "I can't sit here the whole week-end without knowing what's going on."

"Phone the hospital," he suggested, "and see if Dr. Lowry's still there."

"It's 5:30. His office closes at 4:30."

"Give it a try," he insisted. "What have we got to lose?"

*Nothing except my sanity.* But Chris was right. I reached Dr. Lowry in the EEG department as he was going over Jesse's readings.

"Did you see the seizure?" I asked.

"I was just looking at it," he said.

"His eyes went up to the right. Doesn't that mean the seizure originated in the left hemisphere?"

"Well," he said, after a pause, "I'll admit it doesn't look good. But it appears to generalize so quickly it's almost impossible to tell where it originated."

"What are we going to do?" I whimpered. Were we defeated before we began?

"Don't worry about this now," he reassured me. "We've only recorded one seizure. We have to record many more before we can determine if any are originating from the right."

I took a steadying breath. "Okay."

"Remember to reduce his Clobezam to five milligrams, three times a day. And don't worry about the seizure, Nicky. I'll go over the tape again, and we'll see you on Monday."

I worried about that seizure all week-end. On Monday Jesse was hooked up again, and we spent another day watching for a seizure. Dr. Lowry came by later in the afternoon and instructed me to withhold his 4:00 o'clock Clobezam.

I slept on a cot in the hospital that night. Tuesday morning we both woke up early. Jesse had had a good night. So many nights I could have given them, nights so full of seizures the machine wouldn't have been able to keep up. But when we needed to observe them—nothing.

It was Tara's ninth birthday. We had decided to wait until the week-end to celebrate. Tara understood, as always.

The day went by extremely slowly. There was an increase in stomach-aches and shake-outs, but the intense absences and *grande mals* were leaving Jesse alone. When Rita came in to change the tape, she said she thought she'd seen a seizure at 11:57 while I was downstairs having lunch. She couldn't be sure until we were off the machine. Other than that, there was nothing.

At 4:30 Dr. Lowry walked in. "Anything today?" he asked expectantly.

"Nothing yet," I said. "I can't believe it."

"What would you think about taking him off Clobezam tonight?"

"You mean, take him off altogether?"

He nodded. "The telemetry is booked for Monday, and it's the only one in the hospital. I'm sure we'll get seizures eventually, but time is a factor. The other option is to come back in a few weeks."

I shook my head. "If we're going to do this, let's do it now. As long as there's no danger of him going into status and not coming out."

"There's always that chance, even when he's on full medication. But he'll be monitored closely and can be attended immediately if he runs into trouble."

I agreed.

A half-hour later, Jesse's left arm jerked. He turned his head to the left and fell onto the bed. I pushed the button, checked the camera and monitor. I spoke to him as the convulsions began, making sure I was off camera. When Jesse recovered, he began eating his supper again.

When he was finished, I put the side rails on his bed up and gave him his Game Boy. I informed the nurse that I was going for supper. I assumed she would stay with him while I was gone.

I returned a half hour later. As soon as I walked into the room, I knew something had happened. He was alone, in a deep sleep. He didn't wake up when I called his name. I went to the nursing station to ask what kind of seizure he'd had when I was gone.

"He didn't have a seizure," was the reply.

"I'm sure he did," I said. "He's in a deep sleep, and I know he wouldn't be sleeping unless he had a pretty intense seizure."

"I was in there for most of the time," she said, "and there weren't any seizures. Just because he's sleeping doesn't mean he had a seizure."

"With Jesse it does," I insisted

The nurse wrote on the chart: "Approximately 17:35. Mom found patient sleeping in bed and assumed that he had a 'big' seizure because he was sleeping."

When the seizures were later reviewed by Dr. Lowry, he noted in the report: "October 8th, 17:31. The patient was slightly out of camera." There had been no one with him.

I slept again on a cot beside him. Jesse had one more seizure just before midnight, in his sleep. The next day, Wednesday, Jesse was sitting on the edge of his bed and I sat in a chair as we played a game of Crazy Eights on the bed table between us.

"I change it to spades," I said, laying down an eight.

Jesse's arms hit the bottom of the table with a *bang*. The table jerked violently, and hit me as it flipped over. Jesse's cards scattered everywhere, and his body was hurled forward. I barely caught him before he hit the floor. He immediately went into convulsions. I didn't have a proper grip. He was slipping out of my arms. I tried with great difficulty to lift his jerking body onto the bed.

"I need some help!" I shouted, and two nurses hurried into the room.

"What happened?" one asked.

"He flew off the bed and went into convulsions without any warning at all," I said. "I barely caught him."

The other nurse turned him on his side, and Jesse convulsed severely, his head twisted, his face distorted. He made a deep guttural noise with each jerk. All we could do was stand by and watch.

"How can you watch your own child go through this?" one of the nurses asked.

I mistook sympathy for ignorance. "What's the alternative?" I snapped.

"What I meant," she stammered, "was that I would find it very difficult to see my child like this."

"You're right," I apologized. "It would be easier to leave. But I have to be here for him."

Jesse continued to seize for the rest of the day. When he was awake, he had constant stomach-aches, and often headaches after a seizure. The time between was mostly spent sleeping. Chris and Tara came to visit in the evenings, and one day a teacher from Jesse's school came with her husband. Chris and Tara and I were accustomed to visiting while Jesse slept, pausing only to help him through a seizure. I'm not sure how comfortable his visitors felt.

Thursday was much the same. Dr. Lowry came by later in the afternoon and told us Jesse could be discharged the following day. "I think we have plenty of seizures recorded now."

"He's certainly had enough," I said, relieved that we could put him back on his medication. Even so, he continued to seize well into the next day.

Two weeks later we were still anxiously awaiting the decision to proceed with surgery. Finally Dr. Lowry called. "I've finished studying the telemetry tapes and recordings," he said. "I've discussed the findings with Dr. Griebel, and we have come to the conclusion that Jesse should have the operation."

The breath rushed out of me in a *whoosh*. "So all the seizures are originating from the right hemisphere?"

"We believe so," he said. "The ones that involved the left hemisphere generalized so quickly it was impossible to locate their origin. I had been concerned about the interictal activity that seemed to be more prominent over the left hemisphere, but after reading the section on the EEG findings in the book you lent me on Rasmussen's Encephalitis, I realize that many patients have had similar EEGs. The next step is pre-operative neuro-psychological testing, and we'll have to do a Wada test to make sure his speech and memory are served by his right hemisphere."

"When would the surgery be performed?" I asked, cautiously.

"January or February seems to be the best time," he said.

There was still time, then, to change our minds.

That night I re-read all the papers I had on hemispherectomy. I studied the sections of Dr. Andermann's book that I could understand, concentrating on the section on High Dose Steroid Treatment of EPC (*epilepsia partialis continua*). It offered no new hope.

Another section I focused on was "Cortical Resection for Diagnoses and Treatment of Seizures Due to Chronic Encephalitis," written by Dr. Olivier, the Montreal neurosurgeon who had performed the frontal lobectomy on Jesse three years earlier.

I searched for other alternatives. Could we spare the motor strip and delay paralysis? I found my answer when I read:

> Although the syndrome of chronic encephalitis was essentially delineated through surgical efforts to control intractable focal seizures, the indications for and modalities and results of surgery for this disease remain open to discussion. The present study addresses the following points: (a) what is the purpose of surgery: to obtain or confirm a diagnosis, to decrease the seizures, or both; (b) to what extent does the ongoing seizure activity cause the ongoing progressive neurologic deficit; and (c) to what extent can better control of seizure be traded for loss of function? . . .
>
> We conclude that resective surgery is valuable mainly for diagnostic purposes. Cortical resections, even when large, do not lead to seizure control unless hemispherectomies are carried out. . . .

Subtotal hemispherectomy or functional hemispherectomy is likely to bring about satisfactory control of seizures and produce evidence that progression of the disease has been arrested. Whether this type of operation should be considered before the disease has caused maximal deficit remains unclear. It may reduce additional contralateral disturbance due to the frequent seizures but the additional deficit may not be acceptable to the family despite detailed and repeated explanations.

I also studied the effectiveness of *corpus callostomy* (split brain) as a treatment. The procedure was to cut the tissue that transferred information between the two hemispheres, thus stopping the seizures from spreading to the other hemisphere. But that would not apply to Rasmussen's:

> In one sense, the appropriate operation for this disease may depend on the nature of the seizures. It would not be logical to recommend callostomy in a patient with only partial motor or sensory seizures. The patient with frequent secondarily generalized (*grande mal*) seizures, however, may benefit from callostomy.

The frequency of the seizures would not decrease, only the severity of the *grande mal* seizures. The focal seizures—the ones I called "absences," which Jesse had most often —would remain the same in intensity and frequency. In fact, with the reduction or cessation of the generalized seizures, one may expect an increase in intense focal seizures.

In the end, the conclusion was inescapable: hemispherectomy was the only hope we had for saving Jesse from more permanent deterioration. It was our only chance at giving him a future.

I was not totally comfortable with my decision—what parent would be?—but I was more at peace, knowing that I had done all the research I could to come to this decision. I also knew that this decision sprung not only from knowledge, but from love.

*Jo Nanson's neuro-psychological assessment, November 18th, 1991*
On observations of behaviour: In general Jesse's behaviour was very immature for a child of nearly eleven. It would have been more appropriate to a child at kindergarten level.

On grip strength: These results are comparable with the results obtained in Montreal when he was six.

In summary: Jesse is an almost-eleven-year-old boy with Rasmussen's Encephalitis. His neuro-psychological test results are essentially unchanged from those of April 1990. The test results do represent some degree of improvement over November 1990 when he was experiencing a very large number of seizures.

From these results I conclude that Jesse is showing an overall cognitive decline from his premorbid status. He has essentially stabilized since April of 1990. He continues to show evidence of a global encephalopathy. There are some signs localizing this to the right hemisphere but these are primarily present during interictal and postictal states. Other evidence of right-sided pathology includes the poor visual memory. However, there is also evidence of left-sided pathology in terms of the lower verbal than performance IQ, poor performance of tasks of verbal memory, and word-finding difficulties.

I am very concerned about Mrs. Armstrong's expectations for the surgery. I recognize that hemispherectomy is an accepted treatment for Rasmussen's Encephalitis and that it has a reasonably good chance of reducing if not eliminating the seizures. However, I am concerned that Jesse will lose a considerable amount of functioning once his right hemisphere is removed. I am very pessimistic that the functions that are presently served by the right hemisphere will be taken over by the left hemisphere. Both Jesse's age and the degree of left hemisphere pathology that is present at this time make that possibility unlikely in my opinion. I think that Jesse stands to loose a considerable amount of skill for those domains that are normally served by the right hemisphere such as the spatial and affective aspects of language, spatial tasks such as finding his way in space and many arithmetic tasks. In addition he is going to be left with a significant hemiplegia which will require intensive rehabilitation following surgery.

I was surprised by her pessimism. I felt she was failing to take into consideration the fact that the damage to the brain was global, and not confined to the right hemisphere. Jesse's frequent seizures interfered with the functioning of the left hemisphere. After surgery, the bombardment would cease and the left hemisphere could do its work without further interference. The fact that the good hemisphere was already being affected was an even stronger reason to stop the destruction now.

Jo also believed that substantial functioning tissue remained in the right hemisphere. She worried that Jesse might lose more specific right hemisphere functions than simply the motor deficit. She was right, of course, but only up to a point. If we chose the alternative, what would Jesse lose while we waited for the right hemisphere to destroy itself? How much of the left hemisphere would be lost?

Hemispherectomy was not a perfect solution by any means. But it was the best alternative, given our choices. I believed, and still believe, that I was cognizant of all the consequences. If I believed, as Jo Nanson seemed to think I believed, that there was nothing to lose and everything to gain, surely I would not have had such a struggle with the decision.

To be fair, she may have misread my attitude because I was so intent on showing her my point of view. Perhaps I didn't adequately express my concerns and my hesitancy. She was focused on what Jesse would lose; I focused on what he would gain.

# 19 / Jesse's Wish

Doris Newmeyer called from Dr. Lowry's office. "I have some good news," she said in her usual up-beat manner. "I spoke to the co-ordinator of the Children's Wish Foundation, and they'd like to grant Jesse a wish."

"Doris," I whispered, horrified. "He isn't going to die!"

"Of course not," she said. "It's true the Foundation began as an organization to grant wishes to the terminally ill, but for some time now it's been serving all children with high risk or life-threatening illnesses. We thought it would be nice if Jesse could have a wish before his surgery. What do you think?"

Once the shock wore off, I was warmed by her thoughtfulness. "I think that would be wonderful."

"The co-ordinator is Leanne Glover. She'd like to meet with Jesse and you and Chris as soon as it's convenient. I'll give you her number and you can take it from here."

I called Leanne immediately. I warned her that, owing to Jesse's impulsiveness and lack of imagination, he was as likely to wish for a Ninja Turtle as anything else.

"I understand," she said. "First I'll meet with you and your husband so you can give me some idea of Jesse's interests. Then I'll take a walk with Jesse and let him tell me his wish. This will be his wish come true, so we want to make it as special as we can. Some children don't have a specific idea, so we give them suggestions. Sometimes we tell them what other children have wished for. You might give him some ideas. But I want to stress that it's *his* wish, and his alone."

When we spoke to Jesse about it, he asked, "What should I wish for?"

"What would you like to see or do or have more than anything in the world?" I asked.

He thought for a moment. "She can't take my seizures away, right?"

"No, honey, she can't do that. That's what we hope will happen if you have the operation."

He asked again, "What do you think I should wish for?"

I had always made Jesse's decisions. I had always spoken for him. I had never really thought about his lack of independence in that area. Now it occurred to me that I should have been making him think on his own more, make his own decisions. But how can you make appropriate decisions if you're lacking the basic insight necessary to good judgement? Learning to make decisions is part of growing up. Jesse had not been allowed to do that. The disease was robbing him of his childhood without giving him any of the compensations of maturity. Maybe this was a good place to start.

"Some kids have wished for a computer," I said, "or they've wished to see someone who lived far away, like their grandparents. Some kids have wanted to go to Disneyland, or to meet a famous actor or hockey player. It's entirely up to you, Jesse. Think about it, and whatever you choose will be fine. This is your special wish because you're so special."

We met Leanne a few days later. After she had spoken with Chris and me, Jesse and Tara came into the room. Leanne gave them each a teddy bear wearing a "Children's Wish Foundation" t-shirt. Then she took Jesse for a walk. When they returned, Leanne said, "Jesse has decided that for his wish he would like to go to Disneyland. He also said that he hasn't seen his Grandma and Grandpa for a while. So . . . I have a plan. I thought it would be nice if you could go to visit Grandma and Grandpa on your way to Disney World in Florida!"

Jesse was ecstatic. We had told Leanne that Chris's father was having major surgery on December 9th. I'm sure she considered that when she suggested her plan.

Tara was happy for Jesse, and returned his hug.

"You get to come too, Tara!" he said, excitedly.

Her eyes lit up. She looked at Leanne.

"It's for the whole family," she said. "I think you could all use a break."

Chris and I were delighted to see the kids so excited. Happy times had been rare in the past five years. Here was something we could all look forward to. I vowed to put aside all thoughts of surgery while we were gone.

We made arrangements to leave on December 4th and return on the 15th. Since we lived from pay cheque to pay cheque, Chris took out a loan to cover the bills for the two weeks of work he would miss. As for money, food, and lodging on the trip, the Children's Wish Foundation had covered every detail. The family could have a wonderful time without worrying about finances. There are no words to express the gratitude we felt.

Wednesday, December 4th, arrived somewhat more quickly than anyone expected. Our flight left Saskatoon at 8:45 AM. Leanne had requested that we be at the airport by 7:00 so she could meet with us before the flight. Bev had offered to drive us to Saskatoon, so we both set our alarms for 5:30 AM. That would give us an hour to get up and dressed before the thirty-minute drive to the airport.

I awoke in darkness, expecting the alarm to go off at any minute. I turned to the clock. The numerals leapt out at me: 6:10 AM. I jumped out of bed. "Chris! Get up! The alarm didn't go off! Get up, we're going to be late!" I ran down the hall, knocking on doors, yelling, "Get up, Jesse! Get up, Tara! We're late!" The kids woke with a start. "Hurry, hurry!" I urged everyone. "We've only got twenty minutes! Get dressed! Wash!" We had just seen the movie *Home Alone*, and we scurried about with feelings of *déjà-vu*.

The doorbell rang at 6:45. It was Bev, in a panic. Her alarm hadn't gone off! She must have driven like a maniac, for we made it to the airport by 7:05. By 7:50 we were on our way. Chris's parents picked us up in Toronto shortly after noon.

We spent three and a half days with Chris's parents, his sister Jannette, and his nephew Jon-Paul. The Christmas tree was up already, with gifts under it. I wrote my Christmas cards and mailed them from Ontario. We went shopping. We opened presents. We had a traditional Christmas supper with turkey and all the trimmings. We played games. The kids thought it was wonderful. Not only were they having two Christmases this year, but this was their first Christmas ever with Grandma and Grandpa Armstrong. On Sunday we went to the airport, took off our winter coats and boots, and left them with Grandma and Grandpa until we returned six days hence.

In Tampa it was a sunny 82° Fahrenheit. Following Leanne's instructions, we headed to the car rental booth, where we were shown to a mini-van, handed a map of Florida, and told to have a nice holiday. After we had settled into our condo—everything was arranged—we went shopping and swimming and tried to convince ourselves we were actually in Florida!

That night, as I lay in bed, my mind began to wander. Chris was awake beside me. "You know, Chris" I said, "for the past few years I've been promising myself that I would take Jesse to Disneyland some day. And here we are. I want this to be the most wonderful trip for both the kids. God knows, Tara deserves it just as much." A thought struck me: "Do you think Jesse will be able to remember it?"

"We'll take lots of pictures, so he will," Chris said. After a moment, he continued: "I can't help thinking about the surgery."

"We've thought about it for the past three years," I said. "Let's forget about it for a week, and just have a good time."

He agreed, but we both lay awake long into the night.

The next morning, Jesse was up first, anxious to get going. With the threat of a seizure always looming over us, we made sure both kids were beside us at all times. We scrutinized each ride for its "seizure safety," and worked out a backup plan in case one should strike. Usually we managed to go together on the rides, but when there was one Chris's stomach wouldn't tolerate, it was Tara and Jesse and me. We bought both kids an autograph book and chased down each celebrity we spotted, including Eeyore, Pluto, Snow White, Goofy, and Pinocchio. We had a full day, and went back to the condo exhausted.

Chris phoned his mother. His father's surgery had gone well. Now he would have to rest and recover. Chris was relieved to hear the news.

On Tuesday we spent most of the day sightseeing and shopping. After supper Chris took the kids swimming in the outdoor pool while I did some laundry. The kids collapsed soon after they hit the bed.

Wednesday we toured MGM studios. It was impossible to take in all the tours, attractions, rides, and shops in one day, but that didn't stop us from trying! We went to everything the kids were interested in, and the biggest thrill of all was yet to come—Jesse was to meet the Ninja Turtles.

It was 85° Fahrenheit. We were sweltering, but we didn't allow that to dampen our spirits. Jesse had frequent stomach-aches and we stopped often, but we always plodded on. We saw the set of the movie *Beetlejuice* and many of the cars used in particular movies. Chris took pictures of the antique ones. The kids met Darth Vader and had their photograph taken with an Ewok. They also had their photograph taken with characters from *Who Killed Roger Rabbit?* We saw a live performance by the Muppets and got autographs from Miss Piggy, Kermit the Frog, and Fozzy Bear. Tara and I climbed onto the set of *Honey, I Shrunk The Kids*. I tried to convince Jesse to come with us, but he wasn't feeling up to it. His stomach was upset, and he'd been having quite a few small seizures.

Finally we saw the Ninja Turtles. After each performance they handed out autographs and pictures to their waiting fans. We stood with Jesse as he took his place in line. He was wearing his Ninja Turtle shorts and his Ninja Turtle t-shirt. Before we got to the head of the line, though, it was time for them to leave. They wouldn't be performing again for another few hours, and then we would have to wait in line again. Jesse was hot and tired. He had a headache from the seizures, and even though he had come to Disney World especially to see the Turtles, he couldn't wait all that time in line again.

Chris spoke to someone. I don't know how he did it, but he managed to have Jesse meet all four Turtles with April O'Neil just before their next performance. Jesse went into an intense seizure as they drove up, but he came out of it quickly. The Turtles signed his autograph book and then posed with him. He stood there, grinning in bliss, while I snapped pictures. After that he was exhausted, and ready to go back to the condo.

Thursday was Sea World. Jesse had been having frequent stomachaches, so we decided to take in some live shows where we could sit instead of walking in the heat, which he found difficult. We saw the Whale and Dolphin Show, the Sea Lion and Otter Show and Shamu, the famous Killer Whale.

Friday we got an early start and spent a full day and evening at Universal Studios. It was the best day of all. We got more autographs, this time from Yogi Bear, Scooby-Doo, and George Jetson. We saw an animal show starring the ape from the Clint Eastwood movie *Any Which Way But Loose*, and the dogs from *Benji* and *Lassie*. We saw a spectacular show on the set of *Ghostbusters*.

Chris especially enjoyed a 50s-style restaurant called Mel's Drive-in. While he was taking photographs of the restaurant and the vintage cars in front of it, Tara and I spotted Marilyn Monroe strolling down the street.

"Mom, we've got to get Dad!" Tara said.

I agreed.

We chased her down and asked if she would pose with Chris. After he got over the shock, he casually put his arm around her for the picture—definitely the highlight of *his* day! The highlight of mine was a ride on a flight simulator that took us on the same path as the time-travelling wonder-car in *Back to the Future*. We went on a ride adapted from the movie *Earthquake* and several others, including a fabulously terrifying one on the set of *King Kong*. We even got to ride through the sky with *E.T.* The evening ended with a *Miami Vice* night action scene on the water. It ended with a ship blowing up in flames and splitting in half as it sunk.

It was our last day and we all agreed we had saved the best for last.

Saturday morning the kids went for a short swim while I went shopping for a few souvenirs. We were still on a high when we arrived at the airport. We returned the van, had a late lunch, then tried to get our heads out of the clouds while we flew through them.

Chris's mother and his nephew, Jon-Paul, met us in Toronto. Mom Armstrong had prepared another Christmas for us, with more presents and another huge supper. The next day we visited Chris's Dad in the hospital. We were back on the plane that evening. Bev was waiting for us in Saskatoon.

It was ten days before Christmas. We put the tree up as usual, made all the Christmas preparations, but foremost in our minds was Jesse's surgery. I called Dr. Lowry's office early Monday morning. The date for surgery had been set—January 27th. I called friends and relatives to let them know.

A few days later my friend Faye called. She had approached us years ago, before we went to Montreal, about putting on a fund-raiser. I'd been very much against the idea, but now she was asking again. "So many people want to help," she said. "And there's really nothing anyone can do to make things easier for you but offer financial support. This is the only way they can show their concern."

I was still reluctant. "I really don't feel right about it."

"Chris is going to have to take time off work," she persisted, "and there are going to be a lot of added expenses while you're in the hospital. You'll have enough to worry about without worrying about money. We'll keep it small, just the community. Would you think about it?"

I promised I would talk to Chris. "I don't want you to think I don't appreciate it," I said. "It's not that at all. It's just—"

"I know," she interrupted. "You're not used to asking for help. But you're not asking. People want to do this. Give them the opportunity."

I spoke to Chris, explaining it the way Faye had explained it to me. We agreed that we shouldn't stand on our pride. We should be grateful for this selfless and compassionate gesture. We were honoured to have friends like this. I called Faye and told her we would be grateful for whatever she could do. "But, please," I pleaded, "keep it small."

Chris suggested that we look into donating blood before Jesse's surgery. I called the Red Cross to inquire about the procedure, and was told it was against their policy to specify who receives donated blood. "Your son can donate his own blood, however," the man went on, "providing he's well enough to do so. Blood can be kept for a maximum of five weeks, with the last donation a minimum of one week prior to surgery. This would mean that he could donate up to four units before surgery. You can check with his doctor about it."

Doris filled out the appropriate forms.

Christmas at home included my sister Henriette and her children, my mother, my brother Ernie, and his wife Joan. On Christmas Eve we opened the gifts in the flickering glow of the tree. I had asked Ernie to videotape the celebration. We all knew it was the last Christmas that Jesse would be able to use both hands.

Jesse had a *grande mal* on Christmas day, reminding us once again of the fragility of his life. He continued to feel unwell throughout the day. By nightfall he had a high fever. The following morning he had another *grande mal* and wet the bed.

I took him to the hospital, where he was prescribed an antibiotic for an ear infection. He hadn't been eating well since Disney World, and he was losing weight again.

Plans for the benefit were going forward. Faye's husband, Gordon, had contacted Mel Van Dale, a musician in Saskatoon. Mel, in turn, relayed the story to the Country and Western Music Association. They jumped in and asked if they could help. They wanted the benefit held in Saskatoon instead of Vanscoy, because they were sure everyone would want to be involved. Members of the Association offered their time and talents and the Bar-K, a popular country-and-western nightclub, donated their facility. They planned to advertise on radio and television.

"This is going to be *much* bigger than we thought," I said to Chris. We were surprised and nervous about the way the whole idea had taken off. As we discussed it, though, I realized that we were looking at it the wrong way around. I had asked all the doctors and residents I met if they knew about Rasmussen's. I had tried to tell as many people as I could about this disease that no one had heard of, how important it was to get these children diagnosed. Now here was a chance to let a whole gang of sympathetic people know all about Rasmussen's Encephalitis.

I have often wondered how many children are out there with idiopathic seizures, getting worse. How many have Rasmussen's? Because so few doctors have heard of it, they may never be diagnosed. The parents may be searching and never know. They may have to watch their kids seize and seize, develop hemiparesis, watch them deteriorate physically and intellectually, watch their personalities and the essence of their being disintegrate without answers and without hope. Some will not live to be diagnosed. Some will die in status. What a way to have your child leave the earth—seizing to death.

Despite our extreme discomfort about standing in the glare of publicity, we decided to make the most of it.

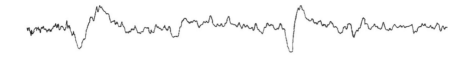

# 20 / The Star of the Bar

Monday, December 30th, Jesse gave his first unit of blood. He went every Monday for four weeks until the operation. As usual, he never complained.

January 6th was our last appointment with Dr. Griebel and Dr. Lowry before Jesse's surgery. I had some pressing questions about the type of hemispherectomy Dr. Griebel would be performing.

There are two types of hemispherectomy. One is termed "anatomical," while the other is referred to as "functional." In the former, the entire hemisphere is removed. It is, anatomically and functionally, a complete hemispherectomy, but there is a thirty-five percent incidence of complications occurring four to twenty-four years post-op. In 1980, in an attempt to protect against these late complications, surgeons at the Montreal Neurological Institute modified the procedure, leaving portions of the frontal and parieto-occipital lobes intact. These were disconnected from the rest of the brain except for the blood supply. According to Dr. Andermann's book, "This functional modification is preferable to the standard anatomically complete operation because it is equally effective in reducing the seizures but protects against the late complications, superficial hemosiderosis, that often follows the latter." I wanted this option for Jesse.

I had also brought copies of a pamphlet, "Hemispherectomy for Seizures," which concentrated on post-operative nursing care. There were sections on the types of procedures, complications, pre-op teaching and counselling, and implications for nursing. I wanted the nurses who would be involved in Jesse's care to read this information prior to surgery. I gave the pamphlets to Dr. Lowry and asked him to distribute them. I then discussed the surgical procedure with Dr. Griebel. I was relieved and reassured when he said he would be performing a functional hemispherectomy.

As I took out some of the other documents I had accumulated on pre-

and post-op therapy for Rasmussen's, Dr. Lowry gave a nod to Dr. Griebel, and they both smiled.

"What?" I asked, suspiciously.

"I don't think you need us." Dr. Lowry laughed. "You have everything covered."

"This is probably the hardest thing Chris and I will ever have to do," I said. "We have only one chance. We have to get it right."

"And we *will* get it right, Nicky. Next question?"

"You'll be anæsthetizing the right hemisphere only for the Wada test?"

"Yes."

I was worried about this procedure. What if he was wrong and speech was not in the dominant left hemisphere? What if I was wrong and the hemisphere wasn't as damaged as I believed? What if there was still a substantial mass of healthy, functioning tissue in there? What if . . . ? What if . . . ?

"May I sit in on the test?"

"Normally, we don't have parents in," said Dr. Lowry. "It can be difficult emotionally. We know what to expect before we perform the test, but it can be disturbing for a parent."

My fear of what I would see was overpowered by my fear of Jesse being alone when he needed me. "I want to be there, Dr. Lowry."

He seemed to sense my need. "I'll arrange to have you present, then."

We covered the other points I was concerned about: post-operative electrotherapy, the probability of aseptic meningitis, other possible complications. When I looked down at my list of things that needed to be addressed at this meeting, every item was checked off. Except one. I looked up again, swallowing nervously. "I have to know one more thing, Dr. Griebel. Do you honestly believe, yourself, that this is the right thing to do?"

He thought a moment, then chose his words carefully. "I deeply regret that Jesse will have a hemiparesis after the surgery," he said, "but I do believe that surgery is his only chance of controlling the seizures. I can only assure you that I could not perform this operation if I did not believe that it was in Jesse's best interest."

I understood his struggle. A doctor is conditioned to cure or repair. "As to diseases," Hippocrates wrote, "make a habit of two things—to help, or at least, to do no harm."

The worst a doctor can do is nothing. The surgeon's job is to repair a deficit, not create one. From a purely physical perspective, Dr. Griebel would clearly be creating a deficit. He had to keep the larger picture in mind at all times. If he lost sight of that, he would be caught in a tailspin.

I nodded. "Okay."

We shook hands, and Chris and I left.

The Benefit for Jesse was in high gear. When it was first announced at the Bar-K, one of the patrons stood up and thumped a five-dollar bill on the table. "This is for Jesse," he declared. Somebody passed a hat and they collected thirty-six dollars. Everyone seemed to be interested in helping, from the Country Music Association to the patrons of the Bar-K to the local media: television, radio, newspapers. It was being billed as the "Jam for Jesse."

The day of the benefit, a Sunday, everyone was up early. We tuned the radio to CJWW, which periodically announced the event. Jesse was looking forward to the "party" that was to be held in his honour, though he didn't say much. He didn't communicate much at all any more. He no longer looked at people who spoke to him, nor did he try to look at people he spoke to. Sometimes, when I did catch his eyes, they looked vacant. I wondered where my boy was, and if I could ever find him again.

Chris and I were extremely nervous—and grateful. We were humbled by the whole experience. If it's more blessed to give than to receive, it's also a lot easier. I had to keep reminding myself that the purpose of the benefit was not only to raise money, but to raise public consciousness about this cruel disease, Rasmussen's Encephalitis.

Jesse looked good in his white tuxedo shirt. I put a black and silver bolo tie around his neck to give him a country look, and completed the outfit with a pair of new black jeans. Tara wore a black shirt, a blue-jean skirt, and a new pair of cowgirl boots. We were all decked out and ready to meet the public. Or so we thought.

We entered Saskatoon just after 2:00 PM. As we neared the Bar-K, we could see the bold black lettering on the billboard:

"JAM FOR JESSE" SUNDAY 2:00–8:00 PM

We tried to find a parking spot, but all the spaces in the lot, the front street, and in all the side streets were full. We were shocked and intimidated. Were all these people here for Jesse? Jesse was anxious to go in. Tara wasn't so sure. Chris and I were definitely apprehensive.

We entered to the sounds of music and chattering, to many familiar faces and many more unfamiliar ones. Aside from virtually everyone we knew from Vanscoy and Saskatoon, there was a truck driver who heard about it on the radio and detoured through the city in order to attend. There were people from Prince Albert who had a child who had undergone brain surgery. The technicians from the EEG department were there.

We mingled, though it soon became apparent that it would be impossible to see and thank everyone. There were literally hundreds of people, adults and children alike. It was often impossible to move through the crowd. People came and went, and there was never an empty seat. Jesse didn't lack for attention. People supplied him with quarters to play the table video games, and he was never without a partner when he wanted to dance.

When CBC television arrived, we went to a room downstairs for the interview. While we were doing that, they held an auction upstairs. Numerous articles had been donated by local businesses and individuals. One man had donated his hand-made guitar. When my sister thanked him for his generosity, he said, "I can always pull another guitar out of the closet, but I can't pull out another little boy."

One half of the Johner Brothers (Brad) arrived unexpectedly. Steve Elliott, the local DJ who was acting as MC, took the opportunity to auction off a dinner date with Brad as well as the T-shirt off his back. Then they called Jesse up to the stage. He stood rather timidly while Steve, whom Jesse had dubbed "Johnny Fever," introduced him to the crowd. Jordan Cook, a nine-year-old blues guitarist, played for Jesse. Ian Eaton was one of the special guest entertainers. As he chatted with Jesse, we saw a caring and gentle person who graced us with his appearance and entertained us with his enormous talent.

We were asked to introduce ourselves and give a speech. I thanked the Bar-K Owners, the Country & Western Music Association, CJWW, the waitresses, the musicians who donated their time and talents, and everyone else I could think of—and of course Faye Sanders who had started it all. "I think God is smiling down on us today," I said, "because there is so much love in this room. I think He's going to watch over Jesse personally on January 27th."

The music and dancing continued. We were overwhelmed by the generosity and compassion of the people, friends and strangers alike, who were there for Jesse and for us. Jesse himself was a zombie by 7:00 o'clock, having overdosed on dancing, video games, and all the attention. Miraculously, it had been a seizure-free day.

The following day our family picture was on the front page of the Saskatoon paper, the *Star Phoenix*. "Boy in need of brain surgery helped by concert benefit," ran the headline. CBC television ran the story on the evening news and again the following day. CJWW radio reported on the success of the jam on Monday and periodically throughout the week.

With all the publicity, it was inevitable that I would get some phone calls. One woman asked if we had tried health foods and herbs. She felt sure that was the answer. A man called to urge us to bring Jesse to his church for a faith healing. I told him we had already tried that. God can create a miracle whenever He wants, I said, but the timing is up to Him. Another woman, under the impression that we were just following doctor's orders, pleaded with me to do more research before having such radical surgery done. She was much more accepting after I explained the many and painful steps that had led us to the decision. I wondered, for a moment, why I was justifying myself to a complete stranger. But I realized two things in short order. First, she was speaking not out of condemnation but out of genuine concern. Second, we had made our private decision public by our own choice. We had no right not to expect opinions, suggestions, and criticism.

When I picked Jesse up at school on Monday to take him to the Red Cross to give his third unit of blood, he walked to the car triumphantly.

"Know what, Mom?" he asked.

"What Jesse?"

"I'm the star of the bar!"

# 21 / Chips in Heaven

Jesse was admitted to hospital at 2:30 PM the day before the Wada test. Although he wasn't going to be on the EEG until the actual time of the test, the leads were attached beforehand. Jo Nanson came up to speak to him, and so did Dr. Nielsen, who was in charge of pædiatric rehabilitation. They brought papers for me to sign. The radiologist, Dr. Denath, came to explain to Jesse what he would be doing tomorrow. Jesse didn't say much, but played with his Game Boy. Chris came with Tara after school and stayed for the evening. Then I prepared Jesse for bed, and we left for the night.

I lay in bed for two hours thinking about the test. The doctors had told me the risks: there was a possibility of a blood clot forming at the site; there was a risk of infection. And this was only a test. How much greater were the risks of surgery?

"Chris, are you sleeping?"

"No." His back was turned to me.

"Are we doing the right thing?"

"It's our only hope," he said, rolling over to face me. "The steroid program's too risky, and for what? Only more deterioration in the end. We either operate now or wait for him to deteriorate more and operate later."

"The responsibility still haunts me. If something goes wrong, could we live with it? I know we're making the best decision we can in the circumstances, but we'll have to be able to live with the results, good or bad. That's something we have to decide now, or we can't go ahead."

I wanted him to tell me, in words I could understand and hold onto, that we would share the responsibility, that we were in this together, that I wasn't the only one making decisions about Jesse's life and future. I knew he hated to talk about it, but tonight I needed some words of wisdom, of comfort.

"I talked to him again about the surgery," I went on. "He says he understands that he'll walk with a limp and that his left arm will be paralysed. He still wants to get rid of the seizures. But I know he doesn't understand it, not all of it. It's so damn complicated. I can hardly understand it myself."

Quietly, Chris said, "I think he understands more than we realize."

I had thought it a blessing that at least Jesse was not cognizant of most of the implications of his disease. For years he had been deteriorating intellectually. His world was becoming more simplistic, more black and white. He lived entirely in the present. When he was feeling well, he acted as if he had never been sick. When he was down with seizures, he waited them out until he was well again. He didn't worry about tomorrow, next week, or next year. He lived only for today.

I remembered a time, about a year ago, when surgery was not yet an option and Jesse was very ill. We were driving home from the hospital when he asked, "Mom, are there chips in heaven?"

I tried not to sound alarmed. "Why do you ask?"

"I don't know." It was his usual response.

Tara was sitting next to me. "He asked Aunty Jeanne what heaven was like about a week ago," she told me. "She said that there were only good things in heaven. All the good things he could think of. Then he asked her if he would have seizures in heaven."

"What did Aunty Jeanne say?"

"She said that Jesse wouldn't have any seizures in heaven, and that I would have two good eyes."

I didn't know if there were chips in heaven. I didn't know what would happen to Jesse next. I didn't know if he would live for another eighty years or if he would die tomorrow. The latter was becoming an ever-greater possibility, or so it seemed. But I didn't want Jesse to be afraid to die. If he thought of heaven, I wanted him to envision God welcoming him with open arms and bags and bags of dill pickle chips.

"Yes," I said, with complete confidence, "there are chips in heaven."

Jesse smiled.

Maybe Chris was right. Maybe Jesse did understand more than we thought.

We dropped Tara off at Bev's at 7:30 the next morning. We were at the hospital by 8:00. The sign above Jesse's bed warning that he was to have "nothing by mouth" had been put up at midnight. On the days he was plagued with stomach-aches he wouldn't have minded. But today he seemed especially hungry. Chris and I tried to distract him as they began to distribute the breakfast trays. We took a walk down the hall.

When we returned, someone had left a tray on his bed table. He went for it.

"All right!" he crowed. "I get breakfast!"

"No Jesse!" I shouted. "Don't touch that tray!" I ran ahead and snatched it away. "It was left by mistake." I took it to a nurse, feeling like Rabbit as he scooped the honey pot away from Pooh and put up a sign: DON'T FEED THE BEAR.

Mike the EEG technician came and checked the wires. Dr. Griebel checked on us shortly before they started the IV in his right hand. An hour later the orderlies lifted him onto the gurney. Chris and I followed as they wheeled him down to X-ray, then Chris left and I went into the operating room with Jesse.

Dr. Lowry and Jo Nanson were already there, along with a colleague who would be assisting with the psychology part of the Wada. It would be from their expert testing and experienced interpretations that the decision would be made whether Jesse's left hemisphere alone was sufficient for basic language and memory functions. It was the final exam on which the surgery would be decided.

Jesse was transferred to another gurney, the X-ray machine looming over him like some incomprehensible beast of lenses and steel. Dr. Denath and his assistant stood by, clothed in green, masks over their noses and mouths. Jesse looked terribly small, but he was relaxed as Dr. Denath explained the procedure once again. Mike set up the EEG and connected the wires from Jesse's head, testing all the connections. Dr. Denath froze the area, then made a small incision in the right femoral artery near the groin.

There were four of us in the small windowed cubicle where the X-ray technician normally stood alone. We watched the monitor as they inserted the catheter. I strained to see through the window. Blood oozed out of the open wound. Several times Dr. Denath asked Jesse if he was all right. Jesse always answered, "Yeah."

I was proud of him. It took courage of a special kind to endure what he had endured. He understood pain, if nothing else.

The catheter inserted, we watched the monitor as the tube found its slow path through his body. It was directed to the right carotid artery which carried the blood supply to the right hemisphere.

That accomplished, Jo Nanson and her colleague stood on either side of Jesse. They administered baseline tests which included naming objects, forward and backward recitation, repetition, comprehension, visual memory, and verbal memory. Jesse managed them all with minimal difficulty. The neuro-psychologists nodded toward Dr. Denath, and he prepared the injection. Jesse was told to raise both arms toward the ceiling. The sodium amytol was injected through the catheter. For a few seconds, both arms stayed up. Then his left arm suddenly dropped to the table with a thud.

I had known this would happen, but I was not prepared for the effect it had on me. My heart jumped. I let out a gasp. Was I mad, allowing this experiment on my son, putting half his brain to sleep? I wanted to go to him. But if I had learned anything through this whole cruel business, it was self-discipline in the face of Jesse's suffering. I looked questioningly at Dr. Lowry. He nodded. Everything was all right.

Jo Nanson called Jesse's name and told him to open his eyes. There was no response. No one seemed worried. I stepped out of the cubicle. Jo continued to call Jesse's name, and the doctors and technicians joined in. Still there was no response. His eyes stayed firmly shut as mine widened. I looked once again for Dr. Lowry. He was studying the EEG and marking it.

*What's wrong?* I wanted to shout.

Just when I thought I couldn't stand it any longer, Jesse opened his eyes.

"Jesse, squeeze my hand," said Jo. Again, nothing. No response. Jesse stared like a newborn baby.

*Come back, Jesse,* I silently pleaded.

His incomprehension seemed to last forever. In fact, it was only two minutes. Then he began to follow simple commands. He was able to recognize and label objects again. They put him through more tests, but I couldn't tell just from watching whether he was "passing" them or not.

"What do you think?" I asked the neurology resident who was standing near me.

"We'll have to wait for neuro-psych to evaluate the procedure and give their results," was all he said.

Dr. Lowry came over. "It seemed to go well, but I'm not experienced in the interpretations. We'll have the results later today."

Jesse had to lie flat for eight hours. A bandage was placed over the incision and checked periodically for bleeding. Dr. Denath came up shortly after the procedure to check on him. He brought a box of chocolates and told him that he had done very well. "In fact," he said, "I'd have to say that Jesse was the best-behaved child I've ever worked with."

His words brought tears to my eyes. I had heard nothing positive about Jesse for years now. It hurt so badly when people told him or me that he wasn't good. I knew he wanted to be, and I wished they could see that.

Dr. Lowry came with the results shortly after 5:00. The neuro-psychologists had concluded that "the right-hemisphere injection did not produce aphasia or significant memory impairment. The left-hemisphere of this boy appears to be sufficient for basic language and memory functioning."

Jesse was kept overnight for observation. Early the following morning,

Tara, Chris, and I went together to bring Jesse home.

With the generosity of the people at the Bar-K—donations were still coming in the mail—Chris would be able to take time off work for Jesse's
hospital stay, and we wouldn't have to worry about bills. When Grandma
and Grandpa Armstrong sent us an additional hundred dollars, we decided
to take the kids to *Beauty and the Beast.*

It was rare that the kids went to a theatre to watch a movie. We usually
waited until we could rent it on video. But that night we spared nothing.
We bought the kids drinks, popcorn, and anything else that might be bad
for them. We enjoyed ourselves thoroughly. I noticed how many little things
we enjoyed more that week, the last week before surgery.

On Monday after school, I took Jesse in for his blood donation, but his
hæmoglobin was down and he wasn't allowed to give any more. I doubted
that three units would be enough,but I had to be satisfied that the majority
of the blood used during the operation would be his own.

As we left the Red Cross for the last time, the nurses all wished him luck.

It was after 3:00 when the telephone rang. I knew it must be the school.
My whole body tensed as I picked up the receiver.

"Jesse just had a *grande mal* seizure," I was told. Pause. Then: "He
doesn't seem to be coming out of it like he usually does."

"I'll be right there."

"Some kids die in status," I remembered a doctor saying. "Sometimes
we just can't bring them out of it."

*No!* I prayed—I demanded—*It cannot end like this!*

I ran into the school. Jesse was in the nurse's room. I was told that he
had come around right after they'd called me.

I was light-headed with relief.

You never get used to it.

I brought Jesse home and helped him onto the couch, then covered him
with a blanket and stroked his hair as he fell asleep. "This is why, honey-
bear," I whispered, "this is why you'll have the surgery."

January 24th was Jesse's birthday, and he was especially anxious to go to
school. He knew they'd be having some sort of party, for it was his teacher's birthday, too, and his last day of school before surgery. I picked him
up at 3:30. His classmates were all calling, "Bye, Jesse!" and, "Good luck,
Jesse!" Mrs. Streisel, the classroom teacher, walked him to the door and
gave him a big hug. Her eyes were shining, and she looked near to tears.
"You get better really soon after your operation," she said. "We're all go-

ing to miss you."

To me, she whispered, "Good luck. We'll be praying for you."

"Thank you," I whispered back.

Nineteen of us celebrated Jesse's eleventh birthday, including most of my family. We all went bowling, then came home for cake and ice cream, and to watch Jesse open his presents. It was a Ninja Turtles birthday. Virtually all his gifts—from colouring books to activity books, from a board game to pyjamas and puzzles—had something to do with the Ninja Turtles. They were all things he could use in the hospital while he was recovering.

I pushed surgery out of my mind for the day. I was getting good at that. I couldn't cancel my worrying, but I could postpone it.

I packed two suitcases for Jesse, one for pyjamas and one for games and activities. I packed one suitcase for Chris and me, and another for Tara, for we had arranged to stay at Ronald McDonald House for a few days.

We arrived at the hospital at 1:00 PM.

The anæsthesiologist came by to introduce himself and ask some questions.

Dr. Griebel came by to discuss the surgery and answer some questions.

"How long will it take?" Chris asked.

"Six to seven hours."

I had to ask one more time: "You're doing a functional hemispherectomy, right?"

"Yes." Dr. Griebel was extremely patient. "The portions that remain will be surgically disconnected and will serve only as a cushion."

"Was my brochure distributed to the nurses?"

"Yes. There's a copy at each of the nursing stations, as well as in the pædiatric intensive care unit."

"They're aware of the probable surgical meningitis?"

"Yes."

Dr. Griebel slowly went through the consent form we were to sign, making sure we understood it in its entirety.

"Can we get progress reports during the operation?" I asked. In Montreal the tension had been excruciating because we'd had no idea how things were going.

"Go to the window at the holding doors. They'll ask me in the OR, then relay it to you. Dr. Lowry will be in and out as well, and I'm sure he will be speaking to you periodically."

"Dr. Griebel, are you worried?"

*Why do I do this?* I thought, even as I asked the question. *What can he say?*

"No, I'm anticipating that everything will go very smoothly. Do you have any more questions?"

I blurted out a couple of unimportant, unrelated queries. I was stalling. I knew it and I suspect he knew it. I didn't want him to leave the room, for that would mean that this phase had ended and the next phase, the surgery, was practically under way.

"If you have any more questions, have the nurse page me," he said.

That eased the transition somewhat.

"Dr. Griebel," Chris said as the doctor was leaving.

He turned, a questioning look in his eyes.

"Please have a good sleep tonight."

He smiled and nodded.

Dr. Lowry dropped in to see if we were prepared, and to see if we had any questions. I didn't think it could be possible ever to be adequately prepared for what was going to happen to our son tomorrow, but I always had questions.

"Are you going to be in the OR?"

"I'll be around the whole time," he said. "I've kept tomorrow open."

Dr. Nielsen came by to reassure us that Jesse would receive active and extensive therapy throughout his recovery. The Binders in Colorado had told me that extensive and prolonged therapy played a major role in the potential of recovery of these kids. I was happy to be reassured that Jesse would be receiving all he would require.

I helped Jesse with his bath, washed his hair, and dried it. Tomorrow it would be gone. I touched his left arm often as I helped him dress, knowing that after tomorrow he would never feel me touch it again.

At 8:00 PM Jesse was given a medication to reduce swelling in addition to his anticonvulsants. We played one last game of cards before we left for the night. We would be back before he was taken to surgery in the morning.

Chris and Tara and I went to our room at Ronald McDonald House. It was after 11:00 when we finally settled Tara down. Chris went downstairs for a while, and I got ready for bed. I turned the reading light on and began to re-read some of the literature I had collected on hemispherectomies.

Tara finally fell asleep. Chris came back just after midnight, and slipped quietly in beside me. He thought I was sleeping. I let him believe I was. There was nothing to discuss. We had to wait until morning.

I wondered if there really were chips in heaven.

# 22 / I Can Sing A Rainbow

I had set the alarm for 6:30, but we were up long before it rang. When we arrived at the hospital at 7:45, Jesse was sitting up in bed with his Game Boy in his left hand and the IV in his right. I sat beside him on the bed, my arm around him. I told him again about the surgery: "Your head might be real sore when you wake up, honey, and you might have a headache. You remember that your left arm and leg will be paralysed when you wake up? I don't want you to be scared, okay?"

"I know, Mom. My leg will come back after a lot of therapy, but not my hand. Right?"

Everything he said sounded as if he were just parroting the words without comprehending their meaning. I would have been happier if he'd cried about it, or told me he was afraid. At least then I'd know that he realized what was happening. But Jesse hadn't cried in years. Sometimes he was happy almost to the point of hysteria. Other times, when he should have been concerned or sad, he was emotionally flat.

I had read that people with left frontal lobe damage were often distraught and depressed, while those with right frontal lobe damage tended to be cheerful and optimistic, with a groundless flightiness about them that bordered on the euphoric. Annoying as it could be at times, I was thankful that Jesse's damage was to the right hemisphere and not the left.

Time was standing still. *Let's get this show on the road,* I thought. The waiting was the hardest thing to bear. Then at 8:30 I heard the wheels of a gurney rolling through the ward, and suddenly time was going too fast. *Not yet! We're not ready yet!*

A man in hospital green came in. "Jesse Armstrong," he said, reading the name above the bed. He checked Jesse's wrist band. "Ready to go for a ride?"

"Yup."

Chris carried Jesse to the gurney. I pushed his IV pole beside them.

My sisters Henriette and Jeanne were waiting by the nursing station with Henriette's husband Eddie and their son Urbie. "There's our boy!" they called.

Suddenly Jesse was excited. He sat up on the gurney and gave each one a hug and a kiss, giggling and squealing.

"Good luck, Jessifer," Henriette said. "Aunty Hen loves you."

"You have a good operation and a good sleep." Jeanne said. "We'll see you when you wake up. Love you, guy."

Chris lifted Tara up to give Jesse a kiss. He grabbed her around the neck and gave her one of his fierce hugs. "Love you, Tara."

"Love you too, Jesse." Her voice didn't waver. "Have a good operation."

The fact that everyone else was holding up helped me to do the same. We all walked with the gurney to the elevator and then down to the basement. Henriette, Ed, Urbie, Jeanne, and Tara went to the OR waiting room. Chris and I continued down the hall to the holding room.

"Hey, Jess, know what?" I asked.

"Love you!" he said, laughing. "Can't get me!"

I ruffled his thick, dark hair. "Darn! I thought for sure I'd catch you this time."

Too soon, they were ready for him. I held his chin in my hand and made sure he was looking at me. "Jesse, I love you very much. You have a good sleep. Dad and I will be here when you wake up." I gave him a hug, and kissed him on the cheek, the forehead, and the nose. I could hardly keep from crying. I was afraid he would die. I was even more afraid that he'd come back only partially, not knowing who we were. I was afraid of him coming back as he sometimes was after a seizure, behind a wall, looking but not seeing, there but unaware.

"Love you, Mom."

Chris bent down and gave Jesse a hug. "Love you, son."

"Love you, too, Dad."

They wheeled him away, and we went down the hall to the waiting room. Dr. Griebel soon appeared in the doorway. "We're ready," he said.

I took a deep breath. "Take good care of him."

He stood there, smiling. He seemed to be stalling. Then he said, "I may not take the whole hemisphere."

I stared at him in disbelief.

"If I see that the tissue looks normal and healthy around the motor strip," he said, "I may leave it connected."

I couldn't believe it. After all the research, the preparation, the anguish over the decision—why was he changing the rules now?

"Dr. Griebel, you can't. They've tried that. It never works. It has to be all or nothing."

I could see he was very troubled. He nodded and said, "I know. We'll see."

The waiting was almost unbearable, especially now that I was no longer sure what Dr. Griebel was going to do. Other people arrived to keep vigil with us: Bev and Shelly, and Shelly's husband Al, good friends all. Jeanne took Tara for a walk. Chris and Eddie went to get coffee at the cafeteria down the hall. At 10:00 Chris went to the window and asked how things were going. Word came back. Things were going fine.

At 11:00 Dr. Lowry came in. "Jesse's doing very well," he said.

Henriette left to teach her class at the university. She returned immediately afterwards. Jeanne continued to go for walks with Tara and keep her occupied. We continued to get progress reports. We continued to watch the clock.

I thought about Jesse lying in that room only yards away. They were taking out half his brain. What would he be when he woke up? Would he be Jesse? *I know we'll never have the Jesse we knew before Rasmussen's took hold. But, please give him back to us as he went in. Don't take any more of him away.* Tears flowed silently down my cheeks. Chris put his arm around my shoulders. I clung to him. I wanted to crawl inside him and feel safe.

"He's going to be okay," he said.

It was what I needed to hear. Bev handed me a tissue. I pulled myself back together.

"Let's go for a smoke, Nicky," Henriette suggested.

I stepped out into the wintry air with Shelly and Henriette. We sat on a bench by the hospital doors. I started to cry again. "What have I done to him?"

"You loved him enough to give him a chance," Shelly said.

"But I'm afraid he's going to die."

I couldn't have said that to Chris. I couldn't have said it to Tara or Jesse. It hurt to say it now, but I felt a sense of relief as the words came out.

"Of course you're worried," Henriette said. "But think what he's survived already. He's going to get through this, too. He's going to be all right."

Dr. Lowry gave us periodic updates throughout the day, and occasionally one of us went to the window by the operating room to inquire further. Time passed extremely slowly. It never occurred to me what it must have been like for the surgeons: on their feet without a break for seven and a half hours, operating on the most intricate and complicated of computers.

At 4:00 PM we were told that they were closing. At 4:15 Dr. Griebel emerged from the operating room, looking tired but composed.

"How is he?" I asked.

"He's fine," Dr. Griebel said. "The operation went well. There were no complications."

"Thank you!" Chris and I said in unison, with a sigh of relief. Then I asked, "Did you do a complete hemispherectomy?"

He nodded. There was regret in his voice as he said, "Yes, I did."

I knew his regret was purely over the loss of Jesse's limb, not over the decision he had made. I regretted the loss too, but I feared the further loss of his mind and soul and physical health more.

"When can we see him?"

"They'll be bringing him by shortly on their way to the pædiatric intensive care unit. You can walk with them. You'll be able to visit once they've settled him in."

"How long before he wakes up?"

"He should be awake within a half-hour."

Chris said, "You must be very tired."

Dr. Griebel smiled and nodded. "I'm going to get something to eat. I'll see you again a little later."

We waited for another fifteen minutes in the hall. Then the sound of footsteps and rolling wheels caught our attention. We walked toward the sound and met the gurney. Jesse looked tiny, helpless. His eyes were closed, his skin pale. His round face looked like a cherub's, except for his mouth which held the tube for the ventilator. His head was wrapped neatly in layers of gauze. A draining tube ran from the back of his skull.

Chris and I babbled together, walking beside the gurney. "Hi, honeybear. . . . Hey bud. . . . Your operation's over, Jesse. . . . You're going to be okay. . . . You did really well. . . . Dad's proud of you. . . ."

Jesse didn't move a muscle.

We followed the gurney into the PICU on the third floor. The others followed us up to the waiting room.

"He looked good," Henriette said, and everyone nodded.

"Yes, he looked pretty good," Chris and I lied.

"Uh-hunh."

"Yes, strong."

"Good."

We were either deep in denial or hallucinating. He didn't look good at all. He looked awful, pale and morbid.

Dr. Lowry came in with Dr. Griebel.

"Is everything all right?" I asked.

"He's resting peacefully," Dr. Lowry said.

"How long till we can see him?" Chris wanted to know.

"They'll call you as soon as they have him settled," Dr. Griebel reassured us.

"How did the brain look?" I asked. With Rasmussen's, it isn't always possible to distinguish the damaged tissue from the normal by sight.

"Some of the tissue was normal in appearance," Dr. Griebel said.

I nodded. I had hoped the entire hemisphere would appear abnormal—an unrealistic expectation, but it would have made it easier to justify the operation.

In twenty minutes they came for us. We scrubbed up and went to his bedside. My eleven-year-old boy looked like a baby. He was naked except for a blue pad around his hips. He lay sleeping on his left side, his face pale and swollen. An octopus of tubes and drains was attached to him: an intravenous tube in his right hand, a device clamped over his thumb to monitor his pulse, a catheter tube, a head drain, leads on his chest to monitor his heart rate, a nasal gastric tube running through his nose into his stomach, and the respirator tube in his mouth. The most alarming tentacle was a line inserted directly into his right jugular vein at the neck. The skin was stitched on either side to keep it in place. The air was filled with the beep of the heart monitor and the hush-whoosh of the respirator.

I took my eyes away from the devices and concentrated on the form on the bed. I gently rubbed his fingers, making sure not to disturb the IV.

"Hi, honey-bear," I whispered.

He didn't move.

"Hey, Jesse. Dad's here," Chris said.

Still there was no response.

The nurse called out to him, "Jesse, Mom and Dad are here. Open your eyes."

My voice grew louder. "Jesse, honey, can you squeeze Mom's hand?"

He showed no sign of consciousness.

"He's still tired from the anæsthetic," the nurse reassured us.

I had to touch his left arm and leg. They felt cold, as I knew they would. Still, I'd hoped they wouldn't. A miracle would have been quite welcome then.

We were allowed to stay only ten minutes at a time.

At 5:45 he still showed no signs of coming out of it. When Dr. Lowry came by, I asked, "When is he going to wake up? Is there something wrong?"

"No, he's fine. It's good for him to sleep. He's been through a lot."

His apparent lack of concern calmed our fears.

By 6:00 o'clock everyone began to head for home. It had been the longest day of our lives. Jeanne and Henriette and Eddie decided to go to Bonanza for supper. They asked if we'd like to join them. We were hesitant at first, but after a moment we agreed it would do us good to get away for an hour. We were unable to eat, though, and after twenty minutes I was anxious to get back. Henriette took Tara for the night, and Chris and I returned to the hospital.

As we passed by the pædiatric intensive care unit, a nurse came out. "Mr. & Mrs. Armstrong, we were paging you. They're going to take Jesse down for a CT scan."

"What's happened?" I demanded, but just then the double doors opened and a gurney with Jesse's inert form on it barrelled through, the neuro resident and the respiratory resident at either end.

"What's wrong?" I demanded again, my voice rising.

"There's nothing to be alarmed about, Mrs. Armstrong. We're a bit concerned that he's still sleeping, and want to make sure he's not bleeding into the cavity. It's purely precautionary."

I was not entirely relieved. I knew the CT equipment was not routinely used after 4:00 or 5:00 PM. We went down with the gurney and sat in the hall outside the CT room and waited. The scan results showed no alarming or unexpected abnormalities.

At 10:30 PM we went back in to see Jesse. He was still unconscious, but no longer totally still. I noticed his muscles twitching. I had expected this, and possibly post-operative seizures as well, but I couldn't help but feel disheartened. I wanted to see his eyes, and caught a glimpse of them when the nurse checked his pupils with her flashlight. They were vacant. He was still far away.

We went back to Ronald McDonald house. I called Faye in Vanscoy and told her that the operation had gone well. I asked her to pass the news on to friends, then joined Chris in bed. We were both extremely tired. Sleep came quickly, but it was fitful. We both woke at the slightest sound.

By 6:30 AM we were up again. We arrived at the hospital at 7:15, but it was 9:30 before we were able to see Jesse. I expected him to be awake by now, but he was still sleeping. We were told that he responded to pain in his right arm and leg. I cringed at the thought of them digging into his fingernails and toenails, as that arrogant resident in Montreal had done. It was a crude way of measuring consciousness, however effective it was.

"Does not respond to commands," the progress notes reported. Nevertheless, he looked much better than he had the previous evening. They'd given him another unit of blood during the night, and his pale skin was showing a touch of pink.

I held his hand, and raised my voice to tell him we were there. I asked him to squeeze my hand . . . and he did! I was ecstatic. "He squeezed it!" I exclaimed, although "squeeze" was a bit of an overstatement. It was more a responsive touch. Still, it was a response to a verbal command, signalling comprehension and acknowledgement. It was the first sign of life we'd seen in him in twenty-four hours.

"Yes, honey," I told him excitedly, "you're going to be okay, Jesse. You're doing really well. You're going to wake up soon. Mom and Dad are waiting for you. I love you, baby."

Although we were not able to visit for more than ten minutes at a time, our visits were frequent. I asked him often to squeeze my hand. Sometimes he did and sometimes he didn't. It was like a metamorphosis, as though he was on the edge of becoming. Sometimes he was nearly conscious, other times he fell deeply back asleep, unable to hear us. I was certain, however, that when I did feel a reaction it was in direct response to my voice.

Sister Emma from our parish came and said a prayer over him. That was when he first opened his eyes. "Jesse, honey, Mom's here!" I said urgently. But I was too late. He was fast asleep again.

At our next visit I read to him, but he didn't open his eyes again. I was becoming increasingly anxious for him to wake up. I asked Dr. Lowry about it, and again he told me that Jesse was doing fine. It was all right for him to sleep.

Our last visit was at 10:00 PM. I read him another book and held his hand, occasionally asking him to squeeze it. His responses were becoming more regular.

"Jesse, can you open your eyes?"

The swollen lids parted slightly, and we had a glimpse of sleepy, hazel eyes. I'd been afraid that he was in pain and unable to tell us. Now I could ask him: "Jesse, are you in pain? If you're hurting, squeeze Mom's hand."

He didn't squeeze it. I was relieved. I wanted him awake and speaking, but it was a comfort to know that he wasn't in pain.

We left the hospital at 10:30, but sleep didn't come easily. After I'd been tossing and turning for a few hours, Chris said, "Why don't you call the hospital?"

Such a simple prescription for peace. I called. Jesse was resting quietly. After that I was able to sleep.

Still, it was a broken sleep. I looked at the clock every time I woke up, hoping it was morning. Finally at 5:30 I couldn't force myself back to sleep any longer. Chris, too, was awake. We tried to take our time showering and getting dressed so we wouldn't arrive too early. By 7:00 AM we were back in the hospital.

Jesse was opening his eyes when they called his name now. He was also squeezing his right hand and moving his right leg when they asked him to. We were able to see him for a few minutes. He squeezed my hand on command, but he wouldn't open his eyes for us.

The nurse was reassuring. He'd been awake for most of the time he was being weighed and given his sponge bath, she said, and he was probably just too tired to open his eyes now. A neuro resident came in to remove the epidural drain. A short time later, he was taken off the respirator.

We weren't able to see him again until 1:00 o'clock, when we were told that he wasn't as arousable as he had been. I asked Tara, who was with us again, if she wanted to see him. She was apprehensive, but said yes.

"Are you sure?"

She nodded.

"Remember what I told you. There are lots of tubes and machinery on him and around him, but he's doing fine. He'll probably be sleeping, but I'm sure he'll be happy to know you're here."

Chris and I took her through the double doors of the PICU, stopping at the sink to scrub up. Tara's eyes were like saucers as she took everything in. We took her to Jesse's bed, and Chris lifted her up so she could see her brother. She didn't say anything.

"Jesse, Tara's here."

Tara took his hand.

"Can you squeeze Tara's hand?"

He could.

"Hi, Jesse," Tara said, her voice breaking. Jesse's right eye opened—the left was swollen shut now—and he looked at Tara for a good thirty seconds. We all moved into his visual field.

"Hey, Jesse!" Chris and I called.

"How you feeling Jesse?" Tara asked.

Then we all started speaking at the same time. "Honey, your operation's over. . . . You did really well, Jesse. . . . Mom and Dad and Tara are all here waiting for you to wake up. . . . I love you honey-bear. . . . You've been having a long sleep, Jesse." Our words ran over and into each other until, slowly, his eye closed.

At 2:00 I was shown how to do his chest physiotherapy with a vibrator. This had to be done frequently to loosen anything in his chest and prevent pneumonia. I was happy to do it, and read him a book when I was finished.

We continued to visit him whenever we could. He continued to sleep. The day was extremely long. We were again reassured by Dr. Lowry and Dr. Griebel that Jesse was just fine. "He just needs more time."

Tara left with Jeanne at 8:00 for the night. At 8:30 Chris went in and started Jesse's physiotherapy. I went in twenty minutes later and took over while Chris went down for a coffee.

"Would you like to give Jesse his bath?" the nurse asked.

I was a bit anxious because of all the tubes and connections, but I wanted to do anything I could to let him know I was there, waiting for him.

I washed him with a warm wet cloth. His left arm and leg were much colder than his right. I washed the sleep out of the corners of his eyes, ever-so-gently around his swollen left eye. When I was finished, I helped the nurse change his linen. Jesse became very agitated when we tried to move him. "Nnooo," he moaned in a voice I didn't recognize. It came from deep inside him. He kicked his right leg, and began flailing about with his arm. His left side remained motionless.

"Ow!" he cried in a hoarse voice. His eyes were open now, but they weren't focusing. He continued to thrash with his right hand.

"Jesse! Honey! It's okay! Mom's here!"

He didn't hear me. The nurse spoke over his cries. "Jesse, we're just changing your bed linen. It will only take a minute."

"Jesse, Jesse!" I called. He kept pulling at the blankets. "Jesse, are you cold? Do you want the blankets on?"

"Yeah," he moaned. His eyes were shut as he tried to pull at his catheter. The nurse moved his hand away. "Jesse, don't pull on that." When the blankets were up, he still took some time settling down. Finally, he went back to sleep.

I was shaken to the core. Everything I had worried about was coming true. The operation hadn't turned out as it had for the other children. He didn't even know who his mother was. I didn't dare ask any questions, for fear of getting answers I couldn't handle. I simply left after he was asleep and went down to the hospital foyer. Chris, Faye, and Shelly were there. I told them that Jesse had woken up and was very agitated. I couldn't tell them he was truly gone, that what I saw in his face and heard in his voice wasn't the Jesse who had gone into surgery three days before.

It was only after Faye and Shelly left that I told Chris what had happened. We both went back up to see him. Jesse was sleeping soundly. I held his hand and told him I loved him. The nurse told us it was common for a patient to be agitated when waking from a coma. I wanted with all my heart to believe her.

We returned to Ronald McDonald house, emotionally drained. We went to bed, but couldn't sleep. At 1:00 AM I heard Chris get up. A few minutes later he returned.

"What did they say?" I asked.

"He's been sleeping peacefully since we left."

The following morning, we weren't able to see Jesse right away. He'd had a good night, but now he was spiking a temperature. His neck and back appeared to be sore, but his head didn't seem to be giving him any discomfort. They believed this was aseptic meningitis, an early complication in most hemispherectomy patients because of the large amount of brain tissue removed. Headache, malaise, nausea, vomiting, and elevated temperature are all common. Daily or every-other-day lumbar punctures to remove twenty to thirty millilitres of cerebrospinal fluid helped to remove the by-products of blood breakdown and reduce the symptoms and duration of the meningitis.

We were able to see him just after 9:00. We went to his bed and called his name. He responded immediately.

"Hi, Jesse," I said, cautiously. "Mom and Dad are here."

"Hey, bud," Chris chimed in. "How're you doing?"

Jesse's left eye was still swollen shut, but his right eye was open and focused. He saw us. His right hand went up in the air, and he waved it around as if he were trying to grasp something. The nurse smiled. "He wants you to hold his hand. He's been doing that for the past few hours, whenever he's awake. I tried to give him a stuffed toy, but that didn't seem to help. He wants you to hold his hand."

I took his hand and held it with all the love I had been waiting to give him for the past seventy-two hours. I relished the touch of him, the response of his hand in mine. I wasn't just touching an unconscious form any more. This was my boy. He was coming back and he was holding on for dear life.

"Hi, honey-bear. You're operation is over. I love you, Jesse."

He didn't say anything. Instead he let go of my hand, wrapped his arm around my neck, and pulled me close for a hug. He held on tight, and I could feel his fever on my cheek. When he finally let go, it was Chris's turn. Jesse pulled him in for a long hug, without a word. We stayed as long as we could, then left feeling relieved, and much more content than we had been when we arrived.

At 11:00 we were told that he would be transferred to the observation unit. Tara was still with Jeanne, but Henriette and Eddy came with us as we walked beside the gurney. They had removed the catheter, and the nasal gastric tube was no longer draining liquid from his stomach. Now it was reconnected to receive oral feeds of baby formula.

The nurses in pædiatrics were pleased to see him back. He cried out when they moved him to the bed; it was extremely painful to his neck and back. Once he was settled, though, the pain seemed to subside. I was about to move a chair close to his bed when I heard him say, in a small, soft voice, "Song."

I wasn't sure I had heard correctly. He had never cared much about music, especially as he became progressively less able to carry a tune.

"What, Jesse?"

"Song," he whispered again.

"You want me to sing a song?"

"Yes. Song."

I put my head close to his. His hand went up, searching. I held it in mine and began to sing to him:

Red and Yellow, Pink and Green,
Purple and Orange and Blue.
I can sing a rainbow, sing a rainbow,
Sing a rainbow, too.

Henriette left to teach her class. Chris and Eddy went for lunch. I was alone with Jesse for a while. I called to him: "Jesse."

His normally big hazel eyes were barely a slit. The left was completely engulfed, and the skin was taking on a yellowish-green hue from the internal bruising. His right eye was beginning the same process.

"Guess what?" I asked, holding my breath.

He didn't hesitate. "Love you," he said in a small, sleepy voice.

I sat up so he wouldn't see the grin on my face, or the tears of pure joy behind my eyes. "Darn," I said. "I really thought I could get you this time. You're too smart for me."

The left side of his mouth remained in its paralysed droop, but the right side went up slightly in an unmistakable Jesse grin.

My boy was back.

## 23 / A Wonderful Grey

The first week of recovery was the most painful. It wasn't the incision or the surgical site that hurt, it was almost everything else. Every joint ached from the meningitis. Changing his bed linen was a torture for him. His temperature shot up to 103° and stayed there. He developed strong and frequent stomach cramps. We dealt with things as best we could: acetaminophen for the fever, a change in food formula for the cramps. Dr. Griebel came in almost every morning to perform a spinal tap to relieve the pressure and check the colour of the fluid. After a week, the central line in Jesse's neck was replaced with an intravenous in his hand, and the leads to the heart monitor were removed. The meningitis persisted for another week.

He spoke a little more each day, but his voice was toneless, almost mechanical. I worried that the cheerful child hidden beneath the disease had been surgically removed along with the right hemisphere. I analysed his every word, testing his memory without making it obvious what I was doing. Then one day he woke up and whispered in my ear, "One point twenty-one gigawatts."

It took me a moment, then: "*Back to the Future?*"

He smiled and nodded. It was his favourite movie.

I'd been testing his memory for a week—discreetly, I thought. Now, with a smile and a nod, he was testing mine.

The people of Vanscoy organized a hockey tournament fund-raiser for us, and the Vanscoy Elementary School held a Valentine's Day pancake breakfast. The students cut out red-coloured hearts which said "My heart is with Jesse." Each person attending the breakfast was given one to pin on. The union members of Agrium Inc. (Potash Operations) took up a collection. The amount raised was matched by the United Steel-workers of America, and this, in turn, was matched by the company. A cheque was presented to us four days after Jesse came home. The *Star Phoenix* ran an update on the outcome of the surgery. CBC television interviewed Dr. Lowry and us, and that night we watched ourselves on the national news. Jesse slept through the broadcast. A large part of his day, still, was taken up by sleep. Some of his relatives hadn't seen him awake since before the surgery.

One day we got a phone call from Ed in Montreal. He had seen us on *The National*. It was good to hear from him, and to know he remembered Jesse. A monk from St. Peter's Abbey in Muenster, Saskatchewan, wrote poems for Jesse; Brother Michael had undergone a hemispherectomy him-self years before. Everyone's support and prayers were deeply felt.

One week post-op, and no seizures. The surgical staples and head band-ages were removed. Once his shaved, swollen head was exposed to the air, he felt cold much of the time. He wanted to keep his head covered, so I wrapped a sheet over his head like a wimple. We called him "Sister Emma."

One morning I walked into Jesse's room from the lounge, where I had spent the night, and he called out, "Notice anything different about me?"

The nasal gastric tube was gone. I congratulated him. From that day Jesse began to eat again. He hasn't stopped yet.

At 10:00 that morning the nurse suggested it might be less painful for Jesse if he weren't in bed while she changed the sheets. She asked me if I wanted to hold him. I was delighted. I hadn't held him in eight days. He winced and moaned from the pain as two nurses carefully lifted him. One supported his swollen head, which seemed too heavy for him to hold up, and the other his body. They placed him gently in my arms. His neck lay in the crook of my arm, and his legs hung over the edge of the chair. His naked, fevered body was hot against me, but he shivered with the sudden cold. I closed my eyes and squeezed him ever so gently, and smiled. I felt at peace—my first-born was in my arms again, and all was right with the world.

In the second week, Jesse had a small seizure. I told Dr. Lowry about it. I knew seizures were to be expected after brain surgery, but I couldn't help worrying. Dr. Lowry assured me it was much too early to worry. Like aseptic meningitis, post-operative seizures were common side-effects. Still, I sensed his regret.

By the end of the second week, the physiotherapist had Jesse sitting up in a wheelchair. A back board extended up to support his head, with a rolled towel around his neck for support. His left arm was put in a sling, and the right carefully positioned so that his IV pole could be pushed be-side him. His left leg extended straight out and was supported at the knee.

At first he could tolerate only a few minutes in the chair, for his fever was still up and his body ached all over.

His voice remained flat and toneless. It was hard to tell what he was feeling. Then one Saturday while Chris and I sat with him, he farted in bed. I teased him about a lion growling under his covers. To our amazement and delight, he burst out laughing. But later that evening, when Chris told my niece Shelly about the incident, Jesse didn't laugh. He began to cry. Real tears streamed down his face.

Chris rushed to his side. "I'm sorry, Jesse. Did I hurt your feelings?"

Jesse nodded, and we were amazed. He had been disinhibited for so long, we'd come to believe he was incapable of embarrassment. It hurt to see him cry, but I couldn't help but feel encouraged by it.

By the third week, the physio was becoming more aggressive. JoAnne, the physiotherapist, put Jesse on a table and strapped down his chest, waist, and legs, then she rotated the table vertically until Jesse was upright. It was the first time he had been upright since before the surgery. Later that week he had more of the same, along with a stretching session. We dreaded those sessions, Jesse and I, as he was still sore and feverish, and he had a constant headache. But we persevered, and they were incorporated into his daily schedule.

By the middle of February, his temperature began to come down, and the colour and pressure of his spinal fluid was almost normal. That Friday we had our first conference with the doctors and therapists. Dr. Griebel attended, and so did Dr. Nielsen, who was in charge of pædiatric rehabilitation. Cameron, the speech therapist, reported that he would be working with Jesse on a daily basis from now on. Rae from occupational therapy told us she would be teaching Jesse how to dress himself. Marilyn, the head nurse, reported that Jesse was still incontinent, and that his needs were about the same as they had been when they moved him out of the observation unit. JoAnne from physiotherapy was unable to attend, but she had reported earlier that she would be working on sitting and pre-sitting skills. She also suggested they start Jesse on pulleys to strengthen his good arm. Dr. Griebel reported that Jesse's condition was stable. There were no unexpected post-operative complications, and his spinal pressure was back to normal.

Chris and I had two concerns: why was moving still painful for him, and why was his voice still so flat? We were told that both these conditions would resolve with time. We left the meeting reassured that Jesse was in good hands and progressing well.

The weekend passed uneventfully. When I arrived at the hospital Monday morning, however, he didn't look well. He'd been up most of the night with pain in his left leg. When I lifted the blankets to look, the leg was obviously swollen. I alerted an intern, who measured the leg and said he would keep an eye on it.

Throughout the day Jesse's leg and foot were extremely painful, and he found it difficult to get through his various therapies. The following day he was given a blood flow test. On Wednesday Dr. Ali, who had been called in to interpret the results, took me aside. He was considerate, choosing his words carefully as he explained the situation to me, then again to Chris who arrived a short time later. Dr. Ali believed that Jesse had a blood clot in his leg, an unusual occurrence in a child. He would have to lie in bed with medication administered intravenously for one week and then orally for at least another two. Dr. Ali's hope was that the clot would either dissolve or attach itself to the wall of the vein. But there was a danger of internal bleeding, he said, because the drugs given to dissolve the clot would inhibit the clotting factor throughout his body, not just in the left leg. The other critical danger was the possibility of the clot moving to the lungs or brain, in which case he would die instantly.

I took God aside for a little chat. I thanked Him again for bringing Jesse through all this. Then I informed Him that I was not going to lose Jesse now. Not to this.

The IV was started that day. Every few hours someone came by to take samples to measure blood consistency. It was a major set-back in Jesse's therapy, but once again we persevered. JoAnne, Rae, and Cameron came to Jesse's room and did what they could for him there.

On February 22nd, Jesse was transferred from Dr. Griebel's care to Dr. Nielsen's. His IV was taken out, and a line to draw blood was inserted into his right hand. A few days later, the swelling in his leg and foot had diminished dramatically.

On February 24th, less than a month after surgery, Jesse moved his paralysed wrist. Then he moved his whole arm from the bed onto his stomach. We were very excited, and I was so proud of him that I made him show everyone who came to visit.

When it came time for Jesse to re-learn to dress himself, it proved to be one of those functions that he lost with his right hemisphere. When Rae put his left arm in his sleeve and told him to pull it up to his shoulder, he pushed it down instead. When he was trying to take his clothes off, the problem was reversed. He was literally "lost in space." With practice, though, the problem seemed to diminish as the function was re-learned by the left hemisphere.

He was confined to bed until March 3rd. Chris went to the hospital early that morning while I stayed home to do a load of laundry. Later, as I went down the long walkway to the hospital foyer, I heard a small voice call out,

"Excuse me, madam." I moved aside, but didn't look around until I heard a familiar giggle. It was Jesse in his wheelchair, with Chris pushing from behind. It was a small incident, but it made his day.

The next day we had our second meeting with the doctors and therapists. Everyone was pleased with Jesse's progress, especially considering the fact that he had been confined to bed for two weeks. He was spending much of his time in the wheelchair, and his days were busy with physio and occupational therapy twice a day, speech therapy once a day, and additional time with the hospital school teacher.

On March 13th we brought Jesse home on a week-end pass. He had been taking a few steps with a cane in therapy, and I was anxious to have him practise this new skill. By the end of the week-end there was a noticeable improvement, and he was anxious to show JoAnne on Monday. He still needed help transferring from wheelchair to bed or toilet. He also needed assistance turning in bed, and he called out a few times in the night for help. He continued to eat and gain weight. He could even tolerate meat now that his stomach wasn't constantly giving him pain. He rather liked it, in fact.

On March 18th we discovered that he could move the fingers of his left hand. With concentration he could squeeze it into a fist. JoAnne used the muscle stimulator to encourage movement. No one knew how much recovery to expect on the left side, so anything he did was a bonus and cause for rejoicing.

Jesse continued to come home on week-end passes, and he was allowed evening passes during the week as long as he was brought back by 8:00 PM. I took him out for supper often, leaving right after his last therapy and returning just in time for curfew.

Chris installed railings on the stairs at home so Jesse would be able to use them independently. He added metal railings to the outside back stairs as well.

Jesse had his own wheelchair now, fitted for him personally. We got a shower chair and armrests for the toilet both to encourage and to ease the transition back to independence.

Unfortunately, as Jesse recovered, his impulsiveness returned. He could stay on task only for short periods of time, and it began to interfere with his therapies. We discussed it at the next conference and decided to restart the Ritalin. The following day, after drug interactions were checked, he was put back on Ritalin. Almost immediately, he began to get more out of his sessions.

On Friday, March 27th, he took a few steps on his own without a cane. I felt more pride in him now, taking his first steps at eleven years old, than I had when he first walked at nine months. "It takes dedication," he said. Simple as that.

As we drove home for the week-end with Jesse and Tara in the back seat, I watched him out of the corner of my eye. He was wearing a baseball cap over his black stubble. He put one of his dill pickle chips on the cap, then he tilted his head toward his sister and said, "Here Tara, have a chip on me."

Dr. Lowry once again expressed his and Dr. Griebel's regret over Jesse's paralysis. He explained to me how the surgery went against everything they'd been taught. Creating a deficit as a result of an error is difficult to live with, but deliberately creating one is unthinkable. I understood him. But I also understood that my Jesse was back, and he was getting better.

On Friday, April 3rd, we took him to his school for Fun Night. He was excited to be back at school, and the kids flocked around him as we pushed his wheelchair through the doors. He stayed home for the week-end, then returned for his final week in the hospital. We spent the last few days saying our good-byes and getting photographs of nurses, residents, doctors, and technicians.

I had wanted to find special thank-you gifts for Jesse's doctors and therapists. I found the perfect gift for Dr. Griebel—an illuminated copy of the Serenity Prayer:

> God, grant me the serenity
> To accept the things I cannot change,
> Courage to change the things I can,
> And the wisdom to know the difference.

It applies to everyone's life, but I found it particularly fitting for a neurosurgeon, especially the one who had performed such a difficult and "unthinkable" operation as Dr. Griebel had performed on Jesse.

Jesse had worked on Dr. Lowry's gift at home the previous week-end. We presented the wooden paper holder to him on April 10th, Jesse's last day in the hospital. In the lid of the holder was a plaque inscribed in Jesse's own printing: "Thank-you for taking away my seizures."

On the trip home we traded jokes. After a brief silence, Jesse piped up, "I made one. What did black say to white?"

"I don't know," said Chris. Tara and I shrugged our shoulders.

Jesse smiled and said, "We make a good grey."

As I laughed, I thought of Jesse without the use of his left arm or leg, Jesse without seizures, Jesse who can think and laugh and enjoy life again.

Things are not always clear-cut.

Some things aren't black or white.

Some things make a wonderful grey.

# 24 / Cheating the Thief

Jesse began attending school again from 9:00 AM to 10:30 AM, but those hours were soon extended to full days. He is able to learn again. He has a lot of catching up to do, but he's making marvellous progress. He responds more quickly, has a much better memory, and is coherent and alert. Reports from the school are positive. They, and we, are delighted with his progress.

Jessse attended physical and occupational therapy twice a week at first, tapering off gradually to once a month, until eventually it was discontinued. We've established a home exercise program, and bought a stationary bike to strengthen his weak left leg in the winter when he cannot be as active outdoors.

The loss of his left field of vision proved to be a problem a month after his discharge from hospital, when he ran into a post that was invisible to his left side. The mishap put him in a leg cast for a few weeks, but he healed well. Gradually the visual field impairment became less of a problem. He has learned, as time goes on, to compensate for it.

Each summer since his operation he has attended Camp Easter Seal, which he loves. The first summer he also attended a program sponsored by the Abilities Council called "Celebrate Summer." Held twice a week through July and August, it offered many different and interesting activities for disabled children, including bowling, crafts, and swimming.

I enrolled him in private swimming lessons (he has his maroon badge now), and in the winter he joins "Snowbounders," a skiing program for the disabled.

Although Jesse's stability and strength had improved greatly by the summer of 1993, he still lacked the balance necessary to ride a bicycle. The Delisle Elks presented him with an adult three-wheeler, for which we were and are extremely grateful. Jesse, of course, is delighted to have "wheels" again.

In 1992 Leanne asked Jesse to be the honourary Chairperson for the Children's Wish Foundation. He was thrilled to attend the opening of the Wish Foundation Home Lottery in the summer of 1992. Then on Boxing Day a local television station did a follow-up on him a year after surgery. In addition, Heartland Productions of Regina produced a half-hour television show on epilepsy in which Jesse and Chris and I were interviewed.

Soon after surgery, Jesse developed brief seizures, which he called "flash movies," in his left ear. They curled the left side of his mouth into a lop-sided smile, then continued down his left arm. These episodes only lasted thirty seconds or so, and they gradually reduced in frequency.

A year after surgery we began to reduce the doses of medication he was on. When the "flash movies" began to increase again, we re-introduced all his anticonvulsants. Then in April 1994, Jesse began taking a new anticonvulsant, Sabril, manufactured by HOECHST MARION ROUSSEL. In December 1995 we again tried to eliminate the anticonvulsants; again the frequency of the seizures increased. We re-introduced the Sabril, and Jesse's seizures now seem to be under control with Sabril alone.

Jesse is currently in grade ten at Delisle Composite School.

We will always wonder why Rasmussen's Encephalitis struck our son, but we have no regrets over our decision to opt for hemispherectomy before hemiparesis. We cannot reverse the deterioration; we cannot bring back what the disease has taken. But early hemispherectomy is one means of cheating the thief, of stopping the final disintegration of our children. It offers a hopeful therapy in an otherwise hopeless situation.

There is life again in my Jesse's eyes.

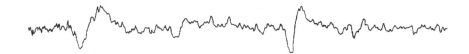

# Suggested Reading

Andermann, Frederick. *Chronic Encephalitis & Epilepsy — Rasmussen's Syndrome*. City: Butterworth-Heinemann.

Bare, Mary A., RN, BS, MSPH. *Hemispherectomy* for Seizures. City: American Association of Neuroscience Nurses.

Freeman, John M., M.D., Eileen P.G. Vining, M.D., and Diana J. Pillas. *Seizures and Epilepsy in Childhood: A Guide for Parents*. Baltimore and London: The Johns Hopkins University Press, 1990. *Second edition available Spring 1997.*

Vining, Eileen P.G., John M. Freeman, Jason Brandt, Benjamin S. Carson, and Sumio Uematsu. "Progressive Unilateral Encephalopathy of Childhood (Rasmussen's Syndrome): A Reappraisal," in *Epilepsia* Vol. 34, No. 4, (1993). The Johns Hopkins Hospital, 600 N. Wolfe St., Baltimore, MD 21287-3141 USA.